THE ULTRAMARATHON GUIDE

A Simple Approach To Running Your First Ultramarathon

By
Michael D'Aulerio

DISCLAIMER

PREFACE

So you want to run an ultramarathon? Congratulations! Deciding to take on such a challenge will not only change your running for the better, but it will change your life.

It's life changing to run far beyond anything you could ever conceive possible. At first, it sure seems like an enormous hurdle to jump. But the truth is, it doesn't have to be as difficult as it may look. Ultrarunning can be so much more than moving your feet forward – or it can be just that: moving your feet forward.

Countless people around the world are surpassing their limits. They do it in different forms and running is by far one of the most popular. In fact, statistics show that over 65 million people in the US call themselves a runner. That's not even considering the rest of the world or people who only run from time to time.

Here's the point: most of us have at least hinted at the fact of running at some point in our lives. Maybe it was to improve our health, or lose weight, or to achieve something more significant in our lives. Regardless of the outcome, running is something that we are all drawn to.

Let's face it, moving is the way of life; it's what we are born to do. Movement unifies pretty much all walks of life, and running is one of the most common forms of movement there is.

Yet, for some, moving is not enough, average running doesn't scratch the surface, and a marathon is only the start. For some, we gravitate toward something MORE. We move towards something greater due to our incredible courage, drive, and determination. That MORE is something called 'ultramarathon running'. An act of running that most trouble to even comprehend, let alone take a shot at.

It's funny how when you tell someone you've run 100 miles, they often reply, "100 miles? I can't even drive that far!"

Sure, ultramarathon running takes a whole lot of physical strength, I know. But the mental strength required is far greater. They say during an ultramarathon you run 50% with your body, while you run the other 50% with your mind. This book will improve both. It will shape your body and your mind for preparing to cross the finish line of an ultramarathon. It will make training simple, prepare you for race day, and teach you the true meaning of mind over matter. It will guide you to the starting line, through the race, across the finish line, and much, MUCH more.

Now, what's the only thing left holding you back?

In your journey to become an ultramarathon runner, you will also face the issue of time constraints. What you'll often say is: "If only I had the time."

Well, guess what? There's plenty of time. And this book will provide you with more of it. *The Ultramarathon Guide* will save you time in your preparation, time in your training, and time in your racing.

Also, you will receive a training program that's easy to follow and simplifies the process. The way it's designed helps you reach ultra distances faster and with far less effort. It will help you to achieve the highest results in the shortest period of time.

And when it's all said and done, this book will not only contribute to improving your running. No, far beyond that. This book will also contribute to improving your life!

I'm referring to the simple fact of pushing yourself to run further, way past your limiting beliefs. A common limiting belief is that the farthest a human being can run at one time is a marathon distance. Well, we will shatter that notion and run farther than ever. You will not only run a farther distance, but you will BECOME the person who can run a farther distance. That kind of change is yours, and it's yours forever. Running an ultramarathon will not only change your life, but it will also rewire your brain.

And the process of becoming an ultrarunner is simpler than you may think. As you'll learn by reading this book, if you keep things simple and focus on both your physical strength and mental strength, anything is possible. You will begin to run farther and be able to achieve any distance imaginable. I tell you this from experience.

At this point, your last barrier will be your own limiting beliefs of finishing. I will help you with this as well. By knowing what to expect, how to train, and that running ultra distances is possible, you'll find the way. Once you finish an ultramarathon, you'll find that it becomes a lifelong passion that you never want to give up on!

It's my passion without a doubt. In life, we all need to grow and progress – this is our human nature. That's why we've advanced from living in caves to flying in a spaceship. The aim of this book is to do just that: grow as a runner and become an ultrarunner. It's to become an ultrarunner, improve as an ultrarunner, and run any distance imaginable. If sharing my knowledge and experiences help only one person reach the finish line, then it has been a success.

I've run many ultramarathons myself. Between races and training runs, I've run close to 100 ultra distances within a 4-year span. Running this much has given me miles and miles of hands-on experience. I went from running a few miles on a treadmill to running 100-mile ultramarathons! One day I could only run across a parking lot, but now, I've run 116 miles across the state of Florida. I dipped my hand in the Gulf of Mexico and didn't stop running until I dipped my hand in the Atlantic Ocean. Not only do I run such long and taxing distances, but I run them through an all-natural lifestyle. No processed foods, no supplements, not even sports drinks. Look, I've run 100 miles weighing 210 lbs and I've run 100 miles weighing 175 lbs, and the differences have been in my diet. I will help you with diet as well. I adapted my body to be able to run over 31 miles at once with no food or water!

Look, I don't speak of myself to impress you – no, far from it. I tell you about my self to press upon you that YES, it's possible and YES, you can do it too!

The best part of ultramarathon running is how we set out to achieve the impossible. It's a direct relation to the flame that burns inside. It's the same flame that burns in you and the same flame that burns in me. It doesn't matter who you are, who you know, or how much money you have. There are no shortcuts. All you have is the motivation that drives you, your running shoes, and 100 miles between you and the finish line. I find this highly inspirational.

So who is this book for? If you are reading this, most likely, this book is for you. It's for those who can feel that flame burning inside and will not ignore it any longer. It's for those who have the urge for something more, for something much, MUCH more. It's for those who will not settle for less anymore and, well, for those who love to run.

This book is for those who are ready to push the envelope. It's for those runners who are ready to step into the ultramarathon world. Finally, it's for the ultramarathon runner who wants to improve NOW.

Look, I've been there. I've been someone who did not run, I've been a marathon runner, and I've been an ultrarunner frustrated ready to give it all up. But I kept pushing and pushing. I pushed through it all, and now that I'm on the other side, it's time to give back. The strength I've gained both on the physical and mental level is incredible, and you can feel this way too!

And here's the best part: I've laid it all out in this book!

So let's get started! Let's dive into each chapter of *The Ultramarathon Guide*. Let's jump in and bring your endurance to super incredible new heights.

It's time to start a journey, a new journey. A brand new journey in becoming an ultramarathon runner!

TABLE OF CONTENTS

INTRODUCTION

Before diving in, let me explain how I made the jump into ultramarathon running. It almost happened by accident. The story starts on marathon race day ...

"My name is Michael D'Aulerio! My name is Michael D'Aulerio!" Screaming this phrase at the top of my lungs was far from helpful as my identity began slipping away.

I stagger-stepped to the side of the road. Race day determination began transforming into confusion and fear. Every step forward was one step closer to complete and utter insanity. Until finally it hit! The worse got even worse; I forgot completely who I was.

I remember thinking to myself, "Is this how the sick feel?" "Is this how insane feel?" "Is this how it feels to have dementia?" I was 20 miles into a marathon, and something beyond hitting the wall occurred.

As I wandered off to the side of the road, I had zero recollection of who I was or what I was doing. I felt lost, lost for words, lost for direction, and lost for reality. When I glanced up at a billboard, the words on the advertisement looked like symbols of some sort. The same symbols appeared on my GPS watch. As I heard the spectators of the marathon beside me, it sounded like they were speaking in gibberish.

Then it happened. I began feeling a warm and dense paralyzing rush through my body. It started down at my feet and began working its way up. First, my legs went paralyzed, slowly forcing me to the ground. As the feeling rose up from

1

my body, I began to lose it! The paralyzing rush then started working its way up through my torso, forcing my body to a lying position. At this point, I could only move my neck.

I raised my head, looking down at my body as I began to develop panicking thoughts to myself. "What is happening to me?" "Why am I losing control of my body?" and "Who the hell am I?" Hundreds of similar questions were racing through my mind at once.

As the warm wave of numbness began to reach my neck, I had no idea what was happening, who I was, or what to do. My neck control was now gone, and I was lying flat on the ground with zero mobility.

When I was on the tipping point of losing any physiological stability I had left, suddenly, it happened. Suddenly, feeling almost faithful, I knew what to do. The moment when your body gives up is the EXACT moment when your heart gives more.

My heart, subconscious mind, spirit – whatever you'd like to call it – knew EXACTLY what to do. In the moment of nothingness, I began purposely developing images of bright lights. My natural instinct was to picture bright lights and to have a positive state of mind. You know, those positive thoughts where you develop a tingling rush phenomenon? Like an emotional sensation gained from achieving something great. Or the feeling you get from a beautiful piece of music.

With zero idea of who I was, somehow I knew positive thinking and heavy breathing was the key to reversing the effect. A natural instinct likely developed from a decade of reading books on health and personal development

Anyway, I began taking deep breaths of fresh air while visualizing big bright lights in the sky. It worked! The paralyzing rush began working its way in the opposite direction. As the feeling began leaving my body, I started remembering who I was. It was the greatest relief of my life!

After spending some time collecting my thoughts, reality began making its way back. My identity returned!

"Wait, I'm a runner and I'm on the sidelines of some sort of race. Hold on, am I running a marathon? Yes, I'm running a marathon!"

I picked myself up with my naturally determined mindset and began moving forward.

With no idea what mile I was on, I began walking. This movement was an unusual feeling. It felt like I had rubber legs on a sheet of ice. There was something off about the connection between my brain to my feet. But it didn't matter; quitting was not an option. I kept moving forward. I pulled myself together and somehow crossed the finish line.

Something happened that day, something that changed my running forever.

Later that day I vomited profusely and had an elevated heart rate for days. For weeks I could not concentrate. Regardless of the adversities, six months later I found myself at the starting line of my next marathon. But something was different this time around. When I crossed the finish line, I felt like I could endure much more.

Why could I run more? Isn't 26.2 miles the limit?

After the race, I went back to tell the man who had introduced me to distance running in the first place. The man who saw something in me and inspired me to run marathons. He began to tell me stories about the world of ultrarunning. He spoke stories of some of the greatest distance runners on planet earth. People who ran across the United States and the Sahara desert. A man who ran 200 plus straight miles without stopping. Runners who shattered 24-hour running records, who run for 6 days, and compete in 100-mile mountain races in the sky. A group of athletes who live outside the realm of athletics.

But it didn't make sense to me at the time. How had I never heard of these extraordinary athletes? Instead of being doubtful or confused about the thought, I began to get excited! I took a long deep breath, and oddly enough, it felt like home. And this was the day I became an ultramarathon runner in my heart.

Within the next 4 years, between races and training runs, I ran close to 100 ultra distances. I've run 50ks, 50 miles, 100ks, 100 miles and longer! I've run 60-mile training runs, 24 hours straight, and 116 miles across the state of Florida. I went from finishing a marathon and feeling like a truck hit me, to running 100-mile ultramarathons with incredible strength.

So how did I do it all in such little time? Well, I began focusing more on my body. I put equal importance on running, recovery, diet, and mental strength.

You see, when training for the last marathon, because of the trauma on my body, I was careful. I had to take it slow, educate myself, and most important, listen to my body. These practices were contradictory to the norm. Instead of listening to the norm, I began listening to myself.

I did things like train on fewer days but running longer mileage, to allow an effective recovery. A more prolonged recovery prevented burnout and injury. Also, I didn't just put anything into my body because another runner or business said to consume it. I found a deeper understanding of running. I finally understood how powerful our mental strength could be.

And here's the BEST part: I share all my knowledge with you in this one book.

So are you ready? Are you excited? I sure am! Let's switch gears and dive right in. First, let's learn exactly what an ultramarathon is.

CHAPTER 1

Ultramarathon?

So what exactly is an ultramarathon? An ultramarathon is any distance longer than the traditional marathon of 26.2 miles. The 50k is the shortest distance. Beyond that are 50 miles, 100k, 100 miles, and even longer! Past these most popular distances, you will find staged and timed events as well. Plus, there are all the distances that fall somewhere in-between them all.

50k

The 50k distance, or 31.06 miles, is a great way to enter the ultra world if you are a marathon runner. Like a marathon, you still feel at home with the fast pace nature, but its distance is longer, so you also get a taste of what pushing the envelope feels like both physically and mentally. Also, fueling can be somewhat the same as a marathon. Most likely, you will apply the traditional gel and sports drink approach if this is how you fuel already. Additionally, there is a relatively large number of 50ks, so it's likely to catch on closer to home. Tired of the same old marathon? Well, try your hand at a 50k ultramarathon. The 50k is an excellent stepping-stone into the ultramarathon world. Then after you finish, you will realize that it's not all that different to a marathon after all.

50-Mile

The 50-mile ultramarathon is almost two full marathons combined. It's both demanding and time-consuming. During the race, you will find yourself running at slower pace and working the aid stations more. Unlike the 50k distance, expect a change in your running dynamics. You will have to compensate for the many adversities presented on race day. But that's what ultrarunning is all about. A marathon is how you perform when everything goes right, but an ultramarathon is how you perform when everything goes wrong. So try and be resourceful!

100k

The 100k distance, or 62.1 miles, is your next option when ready to break away from the 50-mile distance. It's the least popular compared to the rest, with not as many races offered in general. At any rate, it provides you a sneak peek of what it's like to run a 100-mile ultramarathon. The 100k distance pushes you closer to the late hours of the day. The end of a 100k ultra is where the heart of the 100-mile ultra begins.

100-Mile

"When you surpass not the 100km but the 100 miles
mark, that's the point where you show
you are a unique human being."

~ *Yiannis Kouros.*

The 100-mile ultramarathon is where dreams come true. It's an impossible feat for some and a lifetime accomplishment for others. For the mental giants, it's only another notch on the belt. I've run a handful of 100-mile ultramarathons, and they never get any easier. The long distance, sleep deprivation, and pounding on the legs can be devastating. Next, throw in the stomach issues and the mental exhaustion, and you set yourself up for one tough day. But on the flip side, to finish a 100-mile ultramarathon is incomparable. To run a distance that was once thought of as impossible is mind-blowing. Cross the finish line of a marathon and change your life, cross the finish line of a 100-mile ultramarathon and rewire your brain. Every 100-mile distance I've run brought something new out of me that I never knew I had. Completing something you once rationalized as impossible changes your state of mind forever.

Timed

Timed events are also considered ultramarathons. There are 6-hour, 12-hour, and 24-hour races! You will even find 48-hour and 72-hour events as well. One of my favorite ultramarathons I ran was 24 hours. It was motivating to crank out as many miles as possible within a day's time.

There are many benefits to such an event. Your supplies and fuel are always somewhat within reach; however, this can be a gift and a curse. Sure, you have supplies at your immediate disposal which is convenient. But if you become too comfortable, then you may find a chair grabbing your attention more than the trail.

Also, running in a small circle for the entire day can be both physically and mentally exhausting. But it can also be quite the reward, especially when you get to see two sunrises during the same run. In regards to structure, the loops range in size. They typically are between 1-3 miles in length although some races will have longer loops. So enjoy a day of chasing the clock and see how many laps you can run before the clock ticks down to zero.

Multi-staged

Multi-staged ultramarathons can be extraordinarily diverse. This type of race takes multiple days to complete, sometimes lasting 6 or more days in a row. They are overly demanding, as you can't just pack up and go home after a day's worth of running. In like manner, most events take place in unique destinations. You will find races in deserts, mountains, and even across the country. Yes, a handful of runners have run across the United States. Now that's the real definition of "cross country."

All Other Distances

Let's not forget about all the odd distances between the most popular. I've seen a 36-mile race, a 71-mile race, and an 8-hour race. Also, there are ultramarathons over 100 miles. The races over 100 miles may consist of 135 miles, 200 miles, and longer. These are some of the toughest races on the planet!

Ultramarathons are unique in their course layout, elevation, climate, temperature, and distance. Each new race will be so different from the last. It always seems to bring out something within yourself that you never knew you had before. It won't be easy, no not at all, but it will be worth it. So, when race day comes and it's time to leave the starting line, run until it hurts, then ... run some more!

So, now that you've learned what an ultramarathon is, let's jump into the many benefits. Yes, there are benefits to running an ultramarathon! Take a look at the next chapter and see for yourself.

CHAPTER 2:

BeneFITs of Ultrarunning

So you've been bitten by the ultramarathon bug! If you're considering running such a distance, you may have many mixed emotions. I know, it can seem like a huge commitment. Attempting to run ultra-distances can sure be a whole lot to swallow. But the benefits that come along with this amount of running can sure outweigh the stresses. They have, in my own life, without a doubt. If you can make it over the finish line, you will have done something you once considered impossible. Can you imagine what that can do to a person? To achieve the impossible?

It may change your life momentarily, but there's a chance that it will change your life forever. So let's check out some of the most important benefits of running an ultramarathon.

BeneFIT #1: Become Extremely Fit

When training and competing in ultramarathons, you become extremely fit. Miles and miles on your feet will take your body to unbelievable levels of fitness. Add that to a healthy way of eating, and you will lose weight as well. Ultrarunners of all ages run and become built like well-oiled machines. Most elite runners are in their 30s, and runners in their 40s are shattering course records. You might even be fortunate enough to share the trails with someone in their 70s. So, if you train smart and take your health seriously, there's a potential for longevity in the sport. Ultrarunners are built in all different shapes and sizes. The lifestyle change it takes to reach this level of endurance is amazing.

During one race, I was indeed fortunate enough to share the course with a man who was in his 70s. During the pre-race meeting, they dedicated the race to him. They announced his completion of 500 marathons and ultramarathons combined. When you think about it, most individuals who conclude running is unhealthy are those who do not run. It's those who tried running and gave up who give the term "running" a negative connotation.

Look, ultrarunning is tough on the body. After my first ultramarathon, my body felt like it had been pummeled by a truck. I was completely out of commission for a week. But now when I run a 100-mile race on Sunday, I'm back to work on Monday, and in the gym Monday night. The body doesn't know miles; it only knows stress. I'm in the greatest shape of my life, and it's only becoming better. Ultrarunning will do that to a person.

BeneFIT #2: Build Stronger Bones

Along with extreme levels of fitness, ultrarunning will give you stronger bones. When they think of a bone, most people picture a static structure, but actually, bones are dynamic in nature. They are living tissue, and they continuously break down and rebuild. So, as we put more stress on our bodies, our bones grow back stronger to meet their new demands. Ultramarathons put runners on their feet for far longer than average. Prolonged time spent standing promotes a stronger skeletal system – that is, if one makes healthy decisions as well. The point is that we expand by demand, and ultrarunning is one of the most demanding sports there is.

I remember the time I ran a 58-mile training run, preparing for my race across Florida. Approaching 50 miles, I thought to myself, "Wow, I feel incredible." Sure, it was a challenging run, but I was able to keep on moving nonstop for hours. Furthermore, I woke up the following morning and ran 22 miles, totaling 80 miles for the weekend. The strength we develop from ultrarunning does not come from drinking milk, and it sure does not develop overnight. Increasing the strength of our bodies is available to every one of us. When we choose resistance in replace of relaxation, we become stronger, and one way or another we will experience growth.

BeneFIT #3: Create Everlasting Energy

Well, won't ultrarunning make us tired? Of course, but only during and shortly after. But know this: the amount of energy gained in the long run is incredible. The amount of running an ultramarathon requires will send your energy reserves to brand new heights.

Running long distance increases blood circulation and oxygen levels which heightens our awareness. Also, it reduces stress and anxiety which will put you in a better mood and create a better quality of life. All lead to a more energized and vibrant life. And if you become fat adapted, GAME OVER.

The majority of my day, I spend voluntarily on my feet. Momentum is a powerful force as we move throughout our day. If we can move frequently and eat whole foods, then we can gain an increased level of vitality within our bodies. Once an individual gets a taste of a real healthy lifestyle, it's seldom they will ever go back.

BeneFIT #4: Learn to Take Massive Action

Look, there are many physical benefits gained from ultramarathon running – this is obvious. But the mental benefits may be the best of all. When you go through such a rigorous training program and run a distance of such magnitude, it changes your perspective. It provides a fresh perspective on excuses and what you're actually capable of. You will learn to recognize excuses for what they are – excuses – and keep moving forward to race day and any other goal in your life.

In running and in life, taking action is extremely important. You will find this to be most true when something goes wrong, and on race day, something will always go wrong. Take cramping on race day, for instance. When this occurs you could a) lie down and feel sorry for yourself and quit, or b) quickly develop a plan and immediately take action. The choice is yours. Remember, every single action you take both on and off the trail starts with a decision – a decision to try. Your race is YOUR race, and if your action fails, try a new one. You must stay in control of your actions which in turn gives you control of your outcomes. In an ultramarathon, we all want the same basic outcome – to cross the finish line.

BeneFIT #5: Develop Incredible Confidence

Completing an ultramarathon will also increase confidence. After finishing an ultramarathon, you become part of an elite club of athletes. Completing the 100-mile distance puts you close to one in a million – literally. If marathon running puts you in a CLASS of its own, ultrarunning puts you in a WORLD of its own. You may find yourself setting the largest goal of your life and achieving it. That's persistence, that's determination, and yes, that's confidence.

After I finished my last 100-mile race, I never felt better in my life – that is, better after running 100-miles. I called my wife when I reached the finish line with no arrogance or attitude, no, far from it. Humbly and gratefully, I said, "I'm a machine!" Look, although I have a few podium finishes, I'm far from an elite athlete. But here's the thing, my goal has never been about becoming the fastest on the course. My goal has always been to finish each race feeling better physically and mentally then the last one. After this run, I felt like I'd made incredible progress and I say THIS with confidence.

BeneFIT #6: Become Part of an Amazing Community

The community in the ultramarathon world is like no other. Running an ultramarathon places you right smack in the center of a unique community. A community with some of the most passionately driven and uniquely focused individuals to have ever put on a pair of running shoes. No matter what level you reach, there's an incredible amount of support from your fellow runners. We acknowledge each other because we understand from a deeper meaning what it takes. The courage it takes to sign up, the sacrifices it takes to complete the training, and the determination it takes to cross the finish line. Fellow ultrarunners are happy to help, family and friends on the course are delightful, and the volunteers are fantastic.

The ultrarunning community is incredibly supportive. We welcome anyone willing to attempt surpassing their own limitations. Personally, I'm incredibly grateful to share a course with such amazing individuals. Runners of all shapes, sizes, and abilities are out running on the same course to better themselves. The trails do not discriminate. Anyone is welcome, and there's a hidden beauty in this.

BeneFIT #7: Find Faith in the Unknown

Fear strikes when we enter the unknown. When standing at the starting line, we may develop feelings of uncertainty. But entering into the unknown teaches us to have faith. Faith is not something we develop. Faith is something that we all have; it's something we are born with. Faith gives us that amount of certainty to combat hesitation. Sure, we do not know where it comes from. But just like all the most significant historical figures throughout time, you must decide to have it anyway. Ultramarathons will teach you to not only have faith in the unknown but also to have faith in yourself.

Trusting the unknown may be the most beneficial lesson learned from ultrarunning. The benefits not only extend into your running but your life as well. When you have faith in the unknown, you can go after any goal of any size. To believe in the unknown is nothing but a choice and the choice is yours. You can let the unknown scare you or you can let it excite you. You can let the unknown stress you or you can let it intrigue you. You can let the unknown create anxiety or you can let it create curiosity. As I take the starting line of any new distance, I have trust in myself and faith in the unknown. Then I can move forward with excitement to see what I'm made of, but the choice is always yours... so choose faithfully.

Look, running an ultramarathon for the first time will not

provide you with optimum health. In fact, it can be devastating to the body. But for those searching for something more, for those who understand the hidden benefits of suffering, how adversity of any kind is what shapes us and gives us character, for those who can see an obstacle not as an omen but as a challenge to grow, then running an ultramarathon may be for you. It's the human experience in its most natural form. It develops us physically, mentally, and spiritually. If you're reading this book, chances are you are one of these individuals. If so, then on that day, in that race, you do it for one person and one person only. You do it for yourself. You cross that finish line, and you change your life forever.

Now that we know what an ultramarathon is and the benefits that come with it, I will next explain a simple way to train.

CHAPTER 3

Train Simple

"What! I have to run that many miles and that many days!" I know, when you look at an average ultramarathon training schedule, it's overwhelming. But what if you took your training one run at a time? That is, what if you only focused on the mileage of your next run? Suddenly, this enormous goal seems much more attainable. If you can't imagine running a 50k or 100 miles, then break it up. First, imagine running a 5k, then a 10k, then a marathon, and so on. Soon enough, each small achievement becomes one giant success.

Look, there are many different strategies that come along with many different opinions. So, for the sake of running your first ultramarathon distance, I'm going to keep it real simple.

First, the only goal will be to finish. Don't worry about a personal best or how you stack up against the competition. Only have one goal, and one goal only: finishing the race. Do not worry about racing others or how fast you can finish.

I'm telling you, crossing the finish line of an ultramarathon is incredible! A half an hour added or subtracted to your finish time is not going to change how you feel about the big day. It's funny, by not stressing about time, you will likely finish faster anyway. When first-timers race against someone else, they tend to burn out way too early. So remember this: the real race is against yourself.

So, now that you've decided on your race day goal, let's focus on the distance you will run. If this is your first ultramarathon, you are going to run the 50k distance first. If you've already completed a 50k, then move up to the next closest distance. For example, if you've already finished the 50k distance, then train for the 50-mile distance. But for first-time ultrarunners, a 50k will be the best choice, especially if you have a marathon background. It's a much easier transition into the world of ultramarathon running compared to a 50 or 100-mile race.

Also, the differences between a 50k and a marathon are not all that large. So before jumping into the training program, let's discuss those differences. Knowing the differences will be especially beneficial for first-time ultrarunners.

You may be thinking: a 50k, how different is that from a marathon? In layman terms, only about 5 miles, but when you have a limiting belief, it seems much farther. This limiting belief is that 26.2 miles are the most someone can run. But when you drop this thought, the distance goes from appearing light years away to – yes, you guessed it – 5 miles.

When you cross the finish line of a marathon, it feels like it would be impossible to run any farther. But I'm here to tell you farther is an absolute possibility and the 50k is a great place to start.

You will soon come to realize that the 50k distance opens the door to a world full of possibilities. Not only do you break the limiting belief that 26.2 miles is the longest distance runnable, but you gain so much more. You will develop more self-confidence in your running. Suddenly, the real long stuff becomes a possibility – for example, running 100 miles. So to start, let's explore the difference between a marathon and a

50k. After that, I will outline a simple training program. This training program will help make ultramarathon training far less overwhelming. So first, here are the differences between a marathon and a 50k.

Difference #1: Distance

Here's the posing question: is the 50k distance a long marathon or a short ultra? Well, that will depend on the course. As we already discussed, the difference is approximately 5 miles. So, if you're running a flat road 50k, it may seem more like a long marathon where you run at a slower pace and eat more. But most 50k runs are on the trails with many more quick hills and elevation gain than a marathon. On this type, of course, is where you discover the real nature of an ultramarathon.

Difference #2: Terrain

The type of terrain will most likely be the most significant difference of all. One race you may be running up a side of a mountain and the next, quick rigid trails. Going from a city street during a marathon to a technical trail during an ultramarathon is a culture shock. But when prepared, it's absolutely doable. A marathon typically consists of long straightaways, whereas most 50ks have short trails. Shorter stretches create more turns and climbs that are far steeper and faster.

Here's the good news: some 50k ultramarathons are flat. So be sure to view the course description and choose a layout that's comfortable. Here's a word of advice: find a course description that sounds somewhat "doable."

Difference #3: Pace

Your race day pace will change between a marathon and a 50k, especially throughout the last 5 miles of the race. When stepping up into the 50k arena, the most effective and efficient way to pace is to slow it down a bit. For most runners, ultramarathons tend to be less about speed and more about extreme endurance. Still, for most of you, if you go out too fast, then you can expect a vicious payback later in the race. I've been there and done that. You become seduced by the lore of your race day adrenaline, creating one deep hole to dig yourself out of.

Difference #4: Aid Stations

Aid stations vary between a marathon and a 50k, but you know what? They also vary between a 50k and a 50k as well. A marathon aid station typically provides only water, sports drinks, and a few gels. Here you will find a line of volunteers holding out cups to grab and go. You may even catch a volunteer who hands out fruit within a few miles from the finish line. But while running a 50k, and depending on the course, you may find a table or tent filled with food and drinks. However, the more low-key events may require you to bring your own fuel.

Another consideration to take is the length that separates each aid station. During a 50k, the aid stations may be more spread out. That's why runners carry extra fluids in a handheld or worn hydration pack, or similar gear. This type of gear is essential to your 50k race day wardrobe. In like manner, you may need a hydration pack to fill up at aid stations anyway. Many ultramarathons are environmentally friendly as they take place in national parks. So because of the location, they restrict the use of plastic cups to prevent littering.

Difference #5: Gear

Gear also varies between the two distances. As I said before, a handheld pack or hydration backpack will be most beneficial. Gaiters are also a fan favorite in the ultra world. Gaiters connect and cover the upper section of your shoe to prevent any debris from finding its way in. You'd be surprised how much gravel or pieces of sticks your shoe can accumulate without them. A small rock in your shoe at the beginning of a race will feel like a big boulder towards the end. A minor irritation can become a big problem during an ultramarathon. Fortunately, these issues are avoidable with the proper gear.

Difference #6: Mentality

Breaking into an ultrarunning state of mind is essential. Before the point of crossing the finish line of an ultramarathon, we hold many limiting beliefs. As discussed, the largest one that holds us back as runners is that 26.2 miles is the farthest a human being can run. But these beliefs have no physical basis, so try to break up that pattern of thought. To create a new pattern of thinking, you must first destroy the old one – no, not change the pattern, DESTROY the pattern. How can you do this? Become inspired! Do this by reading and watching endurance athletes running unimaginably long distances. By reading this book, you are already on the right path. Your goals become much more realistic when you discover the truth about endurance. When you watch a documentary of someone running across the US, suddenly, that upcoming 50k doesn't seem so intimidating. Remember, even the greatest athletes in the world were once beginners. Your time is NOW.

So, as you see, the differences are not so abundant between a marathon and a 50k. Sure, it takes more time and effort, but isn't that true about anything worth doing in life? Doing what takes little effort will only provide us with small results, it will hardly make us better. But doing what takes more effort will provide us with big results and always make us better.

Since your only goal is to cross the finish line, here is what you are going to do for a creating your training program. First, find the easiest marathon training program for beginners with no more than three runs per week. Also, don't worry too much about time and splits when you train. What's most important is spending the extra time on your feet and covering every single mile. By only focusing on covering the distance, you will avoid forceful extra effort. This way, your body will adapt to higher levels of stress without interference. It will prevent you from quitting due to overtraining, injury, and exhausting. These are all issues you need to avoid as a new ultramarathon runner.

Remember: first, find a very EASY marathon training schedule. The first ultramarathon is about crossing the finish line. You need to build your aerobic capacity and confidence first. Then you can work in your anaerobic capacity and compete. Below is an example of an easy first time marathon training program:

	Sunday	Monday	Tuesday	Wednesday	Thursday	Friday	Saturday
1	Rest	5 Miles	Rest	4 Miles	Rest	Rest	6 Miles
2	Rest	5 Miles	Rest	4 Miles	Rest	Rest	8 Miles
3	Rest	5 Miles	Rest	5 Miles	Rest	Rest	9 Miles
4	Rest	6 Miles	Rest	6 Miles	Rest	Rest	10 Miles
5	Rest	5 Miles	Rest	6 Miles	Rest	Rest	8 Miles
6	Rest	6 Miles	Rest	5 Miles	Rest	Rest	12 Miles
7	Rest	6 Miles	Rest	5 Miles	Rest	Rest	13 Miles
8	Rest	6 Miles	Rest	5 Miles	Rest	Rest	10 Miles
9	Rest	7 Miles	Rest	6 Miles	Rest	Rest	14 Miles
10	Rest	6 Miles	Rest	6 Miles	Rest	Rest	10 Miles
11	Rest	7 Miles	Rest	6 Miles	Rest	Rest	16 Miles
12	Rest	7 Miles	Rest	6 Miles	Rest	Rest	10 Miles
13	Rest	7 Miles	Rest	6 Miles	Rest	Rest	17 Miles
14	Rest	7 Miles	Rest	6 Miles	Rest	Rest	12 Miles
15	Rest	6 Miles	Rest	7 Miles	Rest	Rest	18 Miles
16	Rest	6 Miles	Rest	5 Miles	Rest	Rest	13 Miles
17	Rest	6 Miles	Rest	6 Miles	Rest	Rest	19 Miles
18	Rest	6 Miles	Rest	7 Miles	Rest	Rest	12 Miles
19	Rest	6 Miles	Rest	6 Miles	Rest	Rest	8 Miles
20	Rest	4 Miles	Rest	4 Miles	Rest	Rest	26.2 Miles

So now that you found an easy marathon training program, or have used the one above, let's do some calculations. Let's calculate the difference between a marathon and a 50k ultramarathon. The difference between a full marathon (26.2 miles) and a 50k (31.06 miles) is approximately 17%. So, there's a 17% difference between the marathon and the 50k distance. Now you can apply the difference to your training program. So take each daily mileage from the easy marathon training schedule and increase it by 17%. That's it. For example, if the marathon schedule says to run 6 miles on a Monday, your 50k training run should be 7.02 miles. But to keep things even more straightforward and to make sure you cover the whole distance, round up to the nearest whole number. Instead of running 7.02 miles you would run 8 miles. See below for the newly converted milage which is now your 50k training program.

	Sunday	Monday	Tuesday	Wednesday	Thursday	Friday	Saturday
1	Rest	6 Miles	Rest	5 Miles	Rest	Rest	8 Miles
2	Rest	6 Miles	Rest	5 Miles	Rest	Rest	10 Miles
3	Rest	6 Miles	Rest	6 Miles	Rest	Rest	11 Miles
4	Rest	8 Miles	Rest	8 Miles	Rest	Rest	12 Miles
5	Rest	6 Miles	Rest	8 Miles	Rest	Rest	10 Miles
6	Rest	8 Miles	Rest	6 Miles	Rest	Rest	15 Miles
7	Rest	8 Miles	Rest	6 Miles	Rest	Rest	16 Miles
8	Rest	8 Miles	Rest	6 Miles	Rest	Rest	12 Miles
9	Rest	9 Miles	Rest	8 Miles	Rest	Rest	17 Miles
10	Rest	8 Miles	Rest	8 Miles	Rest	Rest	12 Miles
11	Rest	9 Miles	Rest	8 Miles	Rest	Rest	19 Miles
12	Rest	9 Miles	Rest	8 Miles	Rest	Rest	12 Miles
13	Rest	9 Miles	Rest	8 Miles	Rest	Rest	20 Miles
14	Rest	9 Miles	Rest	8 Miles	Rest	Rest	15 Miles
15	Rest	8 Miles	Rest	9 Miles	Rest	Rest	22 Miles
16	Rest	8 Miles	Rest	6 Miles	Rest	Rest	16 Miles
17	Rest	8 Miles	Rest	8 Miles	Rest	Rest	23 Miles
18	Rest	8 Miles	Rest	9 Miles	Rest	Rest	14 Miles
19	Rest	8 Miles	Rest	8 Miles	Rest	Rest	10 Miles
20	Rest	5 Miles	Rest	5 Miles	Rest	Rest	30.6 Miles

Not so bad, is it? I know – not as overwhelming as other 50k training programs you will find. The best part is this principle applies to almost all other distances. As you can see, the concept is simple, and if you ask me, the simplistic approaches are always the best. So feel free to use this program, or find another and do the calculations yourself. Whatever you do, take this important tip with you: REST days are essential. The longer the distance, the more important recovery becomes.

But REST days do not have to mean REST. When we are not running we can cross-train, take walks, and stand more. But save the leg workouts for your runs. Remember, movement creates more movement, so move all week, even on the days labeled as REST.

How do I know this all works? Well, I've done it myself. When it comes to ultrarunning, rest and recovery are much more critical than most people consider them to be. When you first start off, your body needs extra time to heal, adapt, and grow. Generally speaking, it's a simple process but many times overlooked. It will allow the necessary time to build your aerobic foundation. Aerobic exercise strengthens your heart, lungs, blood vessels, and other aerobic muscles. It will also help prevent common running injuries from overuse. Lastly, and most importantly, it will provide much needed time for your mind to adapt. Your mind needs the time to adapt to the new stresses of running distances farther than a marathon. The extra time off will prevent you from becoming burnt out during training. So remember, rest and recovery are essential, and REST means REST from running, not moving.

So now that you have your training program let's address excuses. Let's tackle the trickiest excuse of them all. The excuse of: "I have no time to train."

CHAPTER 4

Too Busy to Run

When was the last time you wanted to take on a new challenge, but just didn't have the time? I know, sometimes it seems as if it's impossible to find more time in your already busy days. But actually, you have much more time than you may think. The key is to utilize your time efficiently. How much time do you spend getting ready in the morning? At night? Commuting? Watching the television? Cooking? Doing chores? Waiting for appointments? On social media? Surfing the web? Shopping?

The key is to find activities you are spending too much time doing and cut them down. For example, do you watch television every night? Ditch the sitcom, go for your run, and start listening to a podcast from your phone on the way to work. Little changes in your life can save you massive time throughout your day.

Also, before starting a training program, be clear on your outcome. Make sure your goal isn't to just run an ultramarathon. Decide on the distance, know your training schedule, and then begin. When you declare precisely what your goal is, and understand why you want it, you head directly in that path to achieve it. This alone will prevent much wasted time in your training.

I know: ultramarathon training can seem time-consuming. When you are new to ultrarunning, the real challenge becomes finding the time to run than the actual run itself. We all lead busy lives. Between your family, job, activities, engagements, and sleep, it's challenging to find extra time to train. But let's think: you have time to shower and eat every day. You have time for the gym and television every day. If you stop sitting on the couch lost in social media land and instead go get lost on the trails, then you begin to snap out of your lethargic daily routines. You brush your teeth every day because it's a priority and if you make running a priority, then you will always find time to run.

It just takes a commitment and a little creativity. So, want some sure-fire ways to leave the excuses behind and pull yourself towards an ultramarathon finish line? Well, here are some time savers to help.

Time Saver #1: Run Late Into the Night

While the rest of the town is fast asleep, guess what? You've just found the perfect time to run. During the night hours is an excellent time for ultramarathon training. I've set off on training runs at 7:00 pm, reaching home by 2:00 am, and back up at 7:00 am for the work day. That's a 7-hour training run with a full 5 hours of sleep. Sure it's not easy, but neither is an ultramarathon. The night is always available for training.

You might ask yourself, "Won't I be tired?" Most likely at first, but once it becomes a habit your body adjusts. Also, when you run tired at night, your next morning run feels exponentially energized.

So even if it's a run for an hour or two, losing a few hours of sleep is easy to make up during the week. Bedtime is a subjective term to ultrarunners. So have a good night, or should I say good morning?

Time Saver #2: Run Early in the Morning

This time saver is my personal favorite. Try to hit the sack at a decent time and wake up insanely early in the morning. This will allow for a combination of a long run as well as a good night's sleep.

I've forced myself to bed around 7:00 PM to wake up and get out the door by 1:00 AM. This way I've been able to run 30 miles before work or 60 miles at the weekend. Besides having time to train, this is beneficial in two unexpected ways. First, you're not burning up too much of the day. Second, if it's summer, you will cover most of your mileage before the sun rises and temperatures increase. The early mornings are always available – are you?

Time Saver #3: Tuck and Roll on the Way Home

This time saver is my wife's personal favorite. No really, it is. Not able to run because you're going out for the whole day? Next time, bring along your running clothes with you and get dropped off on the way home. Make the drop point the number of miles you wish to run from your house. For example, if you're scheduled for a 10-mile training run, get dropped off 10 miles from your house. There have been countless times I've hopped out of the car while driving home with my wife to sneak a training run in. Are you traveling alone? Thanks to the technology we have today, you can order a car to come pick you up, make a music playlist, and track your run all from the same smartphone. If you look hard enough, you'll always find a time to run.

Time Saver #4: Run to and From Work

We wake up in our square house and drive in our square car only to reach our square office for the day. How about we run some circles to and from work to shake it up a bit? By running to and from work, you fill in the gaps where you'd otherwise be driving. Don't want to run twice in one day? Drive to work, leave your car, run home, and then run back to work the following morning. Not a bad way to get yourself moving before work or to decompress afterward either.

Time Saver #5: Run During Lunch Time

Depending on how long your lunch hour is, you may have time to train during your break. Running at lunch is ideal if you have an hour to eat. Not only does this provide time to train but you will also speed up your metabolism. With a faster metabolism, you burn more calories throughout the day, eat less, and provide more energy to finish the day off. Besides, running will change your mood, and I'm sure your co-workers or employees will thank you for it.

Time Saver #6: Run During the Work Day

Not everyone works a standard nine-to-five job. Some individuals are entrepreneurs, work on the road, or work from home. If this is the case for you, then spend some of your work day running. If you put in a few hours of running into your work day, then make it up on the back end. You might also find yourself to be much more productive after a run. I've made some of my best business calls while on the run. One time I took a job interview from my smartphone while I was running and landed a face-to-face interview. At least when I told them I was a good multitasker I wasn't exaggerating.

Time Saver #7: Run With Your Kids

Running while raising your children can be tricky at times. Most of us want to spend as much time as possible with them, especially if we are busy working most of the time. But if we can give time for ourselves, then we can give more to others, and in this case provide more to our children. Hiring a babysitter for a few hours can do the trick. But if you can't get away from those little rugrats then buy a jogging stroller and hit the streets. They will most likely enjoy it more than you anyway. If a longer run is in need, then bring along some snacks and a movie. It's a win-win for everyone. Your children will be a part of a positive experience, and you will add extra resistance to your training. Why not push them around the neighborhood instead of chasing them around the house?

Time Saver #8: While Running Errands

Need to run a few errands? Throw on your running shoes and get going. Hit the bank, stop by the mailbox, and pick up a few groceries, all on the same run. Sure, you have to stop a few times, but you can treat the stops like your aid stations. Stop, refuel, and start running again. Only a week ago I picked up money for the babysitter and grabbed dinner for the family, all in the same run.

As you can see, there any many ways to make running a priority and to fit it into your busy schedule. Try to see where the opportunity is in your own life and fill in the gaps between other commitments. When you are accustomed to your same old daily routines, it becomes tough to make a change and even tougher to rid of the excuses. Remember, these are only a few unique times to train for an ultramarathon but they are not the only times. If you make running a priority and if you want to finish an ultramarathon bad enough, then the time will be there. The time has been there all along – you just NOW decided to look for it.

So now that you have found time to train, let's sign up for the race. In the next chapter, we will go over what to consider before signing up for an ultramarathon.

CHAPTER 5

Consider This!

Ready to sign up for your first ultramarathon? Or maybe your first race didn't go so well? Whether you are brand new to ultrarunning or ready to step up to the 100-mile distance, there are things to consider before every race. Yes, training is essential, but you must take time to prepare in other ways as well. Ready to prepare? Here are some considerations to make while choosing your race.

Consider Mileage!

First things first, you must decide on the mileage you wish to run and choose a race that meets that goal. When you first begin browsing, you will see 50ks, 50 miles, 100ks, 100 miles, timed, and even longer. But if you're following *The Ultramarathon Guide*, your first distance will be a 50k. Also, once you gain some experience, you may consider strategizing your training with races. I run a few smaller distances like 50 miles or 100k while building up to my big race that I'm training for. Not only does this build up your endurance, but it keeps training fun, fresh, and rewarding.

Consider Dates!

Be sure to pick a date that works best with your schedule. We all have many different commitments in our lives. Sometimes these commitments clash with our running programs. An ultramarathon takes focus, so try to avoid potential conflicts in your schedule. Personally, I finished my first 100-mile ultramarathon while my wife was pregnant with our first. Most days, my training consisted of running back and forth to the store for pickles and ice cream! All jokes aside, I made sure race day was nowhere in sight as we approached our due date.

Keep in mind, some events in our lives are uncontrollable. So, be sure to have a backup race in mind. One time, I ran an ultramarathon with a fever and developed a case of pneumonia from it. Now I know canceling and choosing a replacement race would have been much wiser. We live and learn.

Consider Location!

If you are lucky, then you may locate an event close to home. But for the majority of us, ultramarathon weekend is jam-packed with suitcases and long car rides. Without preparation, you may find yourself hunting for a healthy meal from the local town gas station. Unidentified spinning meat on a heated roller is not exactly what I call a healthy pre-race meal. Also, most ultramarathons take place on trails deep in the woods. Starting a race off the grid creates issues with GPS signals and cell phone reception. Rest assured, there is still plenty of time to post to your social media pages on the way home! So try to navigate the route beforehand. You can even head over early to the race, leaving plenty of time for navigational errors. Viewing directions for the first time on race day morning is risky. This often leads to disorganized rushing and costly pre-race mistakes.

Consider Terrain!

Reviewing the description of the course's terrain is crucial. Is the race going to be in the mountains? If so, you most likely are dealing with high altitudes and elevation. Is the race going to be in a national park? Then you may be preparing for technical trails and many rocks. Are you running along the coast? If so, there are probably flat straightaways with excessive sun exposure. Many ultramarathons occur on some kind of trail, so read up on the terrain so you can prepare.

Consider Elevation!

The elevation is a key factor to consider while choosing between different ultramarathons. Running a comfortable elevation may be the way to go for your race. If not, at least you know what you are up against and can train on a similar elevation. Most race websites will contain an elevation chart of the course. An elevation gain of 30,000 ft. proves to be much more painful in person.

Consider Layout!

Different courses have different distances in different forms. There are point-to-points, out-and-backs, loopy-loops, figure eights, and "where in the world do I go next?" layouts. Know the course layout and reduce the possibility of becoming lost.

Consider Weather!

Weather without a doubt is one of the biggest factors that make or break a runner on race day. I've witnessed this many times. So be sure to consider the time of year and the geographical location in which the race takes place. With this information, you can review the average temperatures and weather patterns. Furthermore, check for record lows and record highs. Sure, you never know what the exact weather conditions will be. Nevertheless, by staying informed, you can plan for the worse. There is always extra room available in a suitcase, and you can always remove layers on the run.

Consider Popularity!

Does the race sell out each year? If so, then be sure to mark the registration date on your calendar. Is there a lottery? If that is the case, you will want to choose a backup race. Also, how many entrants do they allow? The course may be anywhere from packed on a single track to a spread out, small, and low-key event. There is a noticeable difference when running a popular race with 300 runners versus a local one with 10. Whatever size suits you best, the information is always available online.

Consider Rules!

Each ultramarathon has its own set of rules. First, determine if there are any pre-qualifying races required. Fortunately for you on your first ultra, most 50ks have no pre-qualifying races required. But once you begin running the longer races, be sure to keep an eye out. Every 100-mile ultramarathon that I have seen makes it mandatory to have at least one 50-mile race under your belt first. Likewise, for the more difficult ultramarathons, they have specific pre-qualifying races. Furthermore, some of the toughest ultramarathons in the world only accept a resume. Other rules may apply to headphones, headlamps, pacers, and crews.

Consider Aid Stations!

Look at the aid station descriptions and determine what each will stock. Also, it's essential to calculate the mileage between each station. This helps with deciding what gear to bring, what fuel to carry, and what to put in your drop bag. We will discuss drop bags in a future chapter. Additionally, find out what aid stations allow crew members. The event could also be self-supported with zero aid stations. So read descriptions, especially for the longer and more difficult races.

Consider Start Time!

Most ultramarathons start in the morning. The most common time seems to be within the 7:00 am to the 8:00 am range, although there are some that start earlier, later, and even at night. Here's a quick tip: if your start time begins in the dark, you will be required to use a headlamp to start.

Also, there will be a separate time for check-in and bib pickup. Some races have check-in the day before, but most ultramarathons have a time the morning of the race to check in. Furthermore, ultramarathons with multiple distances will have different start times for each. For example, an event may host a 50k, 50-mile, and 100-mile all on the same day.

Focusing solely on the distance without preparing creates one tough day of running. I've been there. It's intimidating to run your first 50-mile race when the hills look like mountains. It's easy to get caught off guard when you're not prepared. But now you know what to consider and what to expect. Remember, preparation is the key to an excellent race day performance.

So, now you have signed up for the race, let's learn how to pack for a successful day of running.

CHAPTER 6

Bring This -> Not That

Now that you've signed up for an ultramarathon, what in the world should you pack? As race day quickly comes upon you, it will be useful to understand what items are essential to bring.

Here's what you need to know: it's going to be a long day, and anything is possible. Ultramarathons consist of extremes. Extreme distances, extreme elevations, and extreme weather conditions. During your first race, you typically learn the hard way why just-in-case packing is so important. Well, luckily for you, since you've stumbled upon *The Ultramarathon Guide*, you will know what to bring along. So let's prepare, be ready, and get to packing!

Bring This → Extra Clothing

When running ultra distances, the day can be long, and the weather will usually change. Various weather conditions on the same day are common during ultramarathons. So be sure to pack extra clothing. Expect to face anything including snow, sleet, rain, and windy conditions. Also, you may encounter plummeting temperatures at night, prolonged sun exposure, and intense humidity. Sometimes, though, you're fortunate enough to catch a perfect day. You never know what you will face until the race begins.

So, with the many possible weather conditions, be sure to pack extra gear. Make sure to bring a raincoat, a hat to block the sun, an extra pair of shoes and socks, and a change of running clothes. Also, if you're not doing so already, you may want to consider compression clothing. It promotes an increase in blood flow and helps prevent chafing and blistering. During the race, layers can always be removed as needed and dropped off at an aid station. Also, you can add extra clothes or any other supplies in a drop bag. This bag will then be dropped off at a particular mile marker that you will have access to later in the race. Have your drop bag prepared, hand it in before your pre-race meeting, and get ready to run.

Bring This → Protection

When running out on a trail or road for hours, your body will need a little maintenance. Extreme weather conditions mixed with continuous motion can lead to many irritations. Most of these irritations can be avoided with a bit of preventative maintenance. First, consider sun exposure. Pack a container of sunblock and consider carrying a small amount with you on race day to reapply as needed. Also, take into account the amount of friction your body will experience. Anywhere your body is rubbing up against itself is vulnerable to chafing. Prolonged running during an ultramarathon causes friction to the body, so be sure to pack an anti-chafing product to apply at the start and throughout the race. One time, my chafing got so bad during a 100-mile race, I ran with a water bottle in one hand and a bottle of baby powder in the other. An ironically symbolic situation for an ultramarathon-running dad. Anti-chafing products can aid in the prevention of blistering as well.

Another issue will be from rocks finding their way into your shoes. Running on even the smallest of pebbles will eventually pierce your skin. To avoid painful feet, bring along a pair of trail running gaiters. As discussed, they attach to your shoes and sit right above your ankles. Gaiters provide a shield from any debris entering into your shoe. Remember, minor irritations at the beginning of a race can turn into major problems by the end. No runner wants to receive a DNF (did not finish) during their first ultramarathon. So be conscious of your body, consider the overall distance, and pack for success. Preparation is the key to a successful race.

Bring This → Electronics

There are various electronics to consider as you prepare for an ultramarathon. If you enjoy listening to music while running, be sure to pack your MP3 player and a set of headphones. Depending on the length of the race, you may want to consider bringing backups. Keep in mind that some ultramarathons do not allow headphones. Be sure to check the race website for details. Most of the time, you will find a disclaimer on headphones for safety purposes. But although they are "discouraged," they are still allowed. Also, look out for the section on headlamps. If a race starts before sunrise or if it's expected to last through the night, then headlamps will be mandatory when the sun is down. Other electronics to consider are a GPS watch, heart rate monitor, or cellphone. Furthermore, with different electronics, remember to bring their proper chargers and extra batteries! Check all power levels before leaving on race day morning. Running in the woods at night with a powerless headlamp will leave you up the creek without a paddle. We all have our own way of running, so bring what works best for you.

Bring This → Fuel

Finally, you will want to consider your fueling technique as well as what fuel to pack. Find out what's going to be provided at the aid stations. If your fuel of choice will not be available, then pack your preferred food, gels, or electrolytes. Aid stations are filled with food, water, and sports drinks.

Also, consider what hydration gear to use for fueling. It will most likely be a handheld water bottle or some type of hydration backpack. This hydration gear will consist of containers for fluid and pockets for fuel. Also, consider the quality of your hydration gear; you must rely on it to fuel you through many miles. Make sure to bring one you can depend on.

When running ultramarathons, you learn a lot about running and, at the same time, you learn a lot about yourself. While spending so much time on long runs, you will begin to notice what is beneficial for you. With each new race, you can take this packing list and fine-tune it to meet your personal needs. Work in congruence with your crew or with your pacer and pack for an incredible day of running. Ultramarathon race day is a transformative day, a day you will come to realize what you are truly capable of: anything that you set your mind to... oh, and anything you pack for!

Now that you are packed and ready to go, let's discuss what to expect on race day morning.

CHAPTER 7

Rest, Rise, and Run

Ultramarathon race day morning can take several turns, so let's prepare and focus. I've taken the starting line with ease, and I've taken the starting line with a shirt on backward and a grumbling stomach. But with preparation, it can be smooth and even leveraged to your advantage. Race day can fly by quickly, or it can fly by YOU. So here's some morning guidance that will help you reach the starting line stress-free and focused on your run.

Morning Guidance #1: Have Your Clothes Ready

For race day morning, try laying out your clothes and having your bags packed, ready to go. Preparation will reduce stress, wasted time, and the chances of forgetting any gear. Attempting to put your things together last minute will only lead to wasted energy. This same wasted energy could be used for running in the race. So, by setting time aside the night before to pack, you increase the odds of a good night's sleep and a good morning start.

Morning Guidance #2: Have Breakfast Planned

Most runners will have their meal planned out for the morning. If you enjoy a hot meal and are staying at a hotel, then be sure to confirm their breakfast time. If you prefer a quick snack, then have your meal replacement bars with you. Also, if you are a coffee or tea drinker, then find out who's brewing in the morning. Personally, for my own nutritional reasoning, I take the starting line on an empty stomach. But whatever your strategy may be, it's best to stay clear of trying anything new, the morning of.

Morning Guidance #3: Print Directions

When navigating to the starting line, it's best to have the address on your GPS as well as a set of printed directions. Most ultramarathons take place in areas with little to no GPS signal or cell phone reception. When signals are lost, it's beneficial to have a set of printed directions handy. If possible, drive to the starting line the night before. A printed set of directions will assist in eliminating any wasted time on the morning of the race. Rushing to the starting line will only cause unwarranted mistakes and wasted energy.

Morning Guidance #4: Know Bib Pickup Time

Before every ultramarathon, there is usually a period dedicated to picking up your bib. For those who don't know, a "bib" is your race number which is safety pinned to your clothing. Your bib identifies who you are on the course. It usually contains a sensor that monitors when you cross both the start line and the finish line. All in all, bib pickup is straightforward, and you will receive a pretty awesome race shirt too.

Morning Guidance #5: Bathroom Lines Take Time

Most ultramarathon mornings consist of standing in line for the bathroom. Yes, there are far fewer people who take part in an ultramarathon compared to a big city marathon; however, there are fewer bathrooms. So when it's all said and done, the ratio can be quite similar. How you work the bathroom lines on race day morning is an art form. It will all come down to timing, and if all else fails, there's rarely ever a line for the bushes.

Morning Guidance #6: Pack a Drop Bag

As discussed, a drop bag is for extra supplies which are then "dropped" at a particular aid station. Fuel refills, extra clothes, and useful supplies are some of the things found in such a bag. This bag can then be handed in on race day morning. So, drop everything and get that drop bag ready!

Morning Guidance #7: Conduct a Mental Checklist

Have your mental checklist ready for race day morning. Write it down, if need be. I typically start at my feet and work my way up. Shoes, compression socks, gaiters, running shorts, compression shorts, handhelds, iPods, headphones, sunblock, petroleum jelly, hat, and so on. This checklist eventually becomes fine-tuned to your requirements. After a few races, it becomes routine. Running through your checklist will only take a minute but will save you from much grief. It avoids that gut-wrenching feeling during a race when you realize something significant was left behind.

Morning Guidance #8: Remember the Small Things

There are many small things to remind yourself of on race day morning. Sometimes the most minor things can have the most substantial impact on your performance. Some examples are filling up your hydration gear, packing enough fuel, applying an anti-chafing product, and checking the battery life of your headlamp. So try to keep things simple and remember the small things to avoid the large problems.

Morning Guidance #9: Listen to the Race Announcements

Before each ultramarathon, there will be a pre-race announcement. It typically takes place 10-15 minutes before the start. The race director will review the rules, the course, and thank the volunteers. What you want to pay especially close attention to is in regards to the course and any revisions made. Listening to music through a pre-race announcement may cost you extra mileage. If you miss an announcement on a course change, then you could run the wrong way or even get lost.

Morning Guidance #10: The Countdown is Powerful

30 seconds to go! It's time to take it all in. Months and miles of training rush through your mind, all packaged into a 30-second countdown. Think back on those sleepless nights, frigid cold mornings, and weekend sacrifices. Think back on those incredible runs that built your confidence and those not-so-incredible ones that built your strength. Think back to those sore legs you've walked around with for months. You earned this; this race is yours, and it's finally about to begin. After 30 seconds, suddenly, all your training becomes a distant memory. It's now time to leave the past behind and shift your mindset to the present – and in the present, there's only one thing left to do... run!

Wow, race day morning sure flew by! Now that the race has begun, I will provide you with some tips on running and reaching the finish line.

CHAPTER 8

Cross the Finish Line

You're doing it! You're running your first ultramarathon! Let's hurry and dive into some helpful tips to get you across that finish line. I cannot deny that mechanics are an essential part of completing an ultramarathon, so I will touch on some mechanics. But here's the thing, if you already have some basic mechanics down, then you can focus on what's most important. You can focus on what gets you from the couch to the trail and what transforms you from running a 10-mile race to a 100-mile ultramarathon. This focus is psychological. This focus is your mental strength. It's your mental strength that keeps your legs moving when the body tries shutting down. It's your mental strength that pushes you through those last few endless miles to the finish. It's your mental strength that tells you to push harder and go farther than ever before. So if you haven't done so yet, let's start with how you get to the finish line.

Helpful Tip #1: Get to the Starting Line

We often fail before we ever begin. I'd say most of the time, it's from focusing on fears we've created from thin air. For example, causes of failure or being unworthy. But what's incredible about becoming a runner is that it literally ONLY means taking one step forward, and poof – you're a runner. However, we naturally develop excuses during training to stop us from even getting to the starting line. Discussing your excuses with someone else will never help. It only provides more comfort to quit before you even start. Friends and loved ones mean well, they really do. But, unfortunately, it's difficult to make logical sense out of running an ultramarathon. So, try and recognize excuses for what they are – excuses – and keep moving forward to race day. Because there's one thing I know for sure: if you look for excuses, you will always find them. Remember, there's no such thing as bad weather, only bad gear!

Helpful Tip #2: Have Absolute Certainty

Have absolute certainty for getting to the starting line and crossing the finish. When building up to race day, eliminate any thoughts of not finishing. This type of mentality is controllable. But just as easily as you can control this, you can just as easily lose control. If you want to complete your first ultramarathon bad enough, then you can do it! The secret ingredient is FOCUS. Make a clear and precise decision. I ran my first ultramarathon four years ago. Since then, between races and training runs, I've run nearly 100 ultra-distances. Before race day, I make sure I'm absolutely certain that I will cross the finish line. In training, I run so far away from home that I must complete the run unless I want to hitchhike my way back. One time, during a training run, I was breaking my 50k time approximately 15 miles from my house when I hurt my knee. What a long walk home that was!

Helpful Tip #3: Stay Calm and Hold On

When the race begins, it's common to get a rush of adrenaline and you may not even realize it. This causes a much quicker starting pace. If you give in to this urge, it will undoubtedly catch up with you later in the race. Remind yourself of this rush at the starting line. Try to stay in tune with your body and back off your pace slightly. Personally, I do not wear watches on race day. I run on feeling. From experience, I'm usually able to notice the difference between an adrenaline pace versus a race day groove – usually!

During one of my first races ever, I noticed a super-excited guy running next to me. He was smiling, waving to all the bystanders, and jumping around for a number of miles. I remember thinking to myself, "I hope he's conserving some of that energy." Up by mile 16, I saw the same super-excited guy lying flat on his back on the side of the road. He, unfortunately, dropped out.

Helpful Tip #4: Run Your Own Race

There are many runners of all different shapes, sizes, and speeds. Try not to get caught up in attempting to run faster than the person next to you. It's a long race, and this common mistake can cost you a high amount of energy too soon. It's a tough and lonely place to be out of energy on your 30th mile with 20 miles to go. Or your 45th mile with 65 miles to go. I know this from experience. The real race is against yourself. Let your internal control affect your external environment, not the other way around.

Helpful Tip #5: Same Fueling Technique

It's a good idea on race day to fuel the same way you've fueled during training. I seldom ever try something new on race day. I've learned the harm from this first hand. Race day is not the day for experimentation.

One time during a race, before I started all-natural fueling, I used whatever was at the aid stations. Between this, the heat, and hydration issues, I pushed myself to a point where I lost full body control. I forgot who I was! I couldn't tell you my name or what I was doing. Somehow I found a way to finish, but it was dangerously difficult. Also, it took several days to get me back to normal. This would be a worst-case scenario, but the point is to be careful and stick to the plan.

Helpful Tip #6: Know Your Aid Stations

Most races will have a section on their website dedicated to aid stations. Here you will find information on the food, drinks, and locations. If you have any more questions, you can always email the race director. This information will allow you to plan what fuel to carry and what to leave home. Our bodies are all different. A fueling plan for one person could be entirely different for another. There's no right or wrong way to do it. Find out what works best for you. Personally, I prefer almond butter, dried fruit, and a handheld filled with coconut water.

Helpful Tip #7: Uphill Strides Small and Quick

Keep your uphill strides small and quick. Think about it – if you put a pair of weights in your hands and walk uphill, what's easier? To lunge or to take quick, short steps? Hills can be a great change of pace and a chance for different muscles to be activated. Hills can be your best friend or your worst friend; the choice is yours.

Helpful Tip #8: Stay in the Present

While racing, try not to think about the finish line. I've been a quarter mile away from the finish line when it felt like an eternity and I've been 30 miles away from the finish line when it felt like a walk in the park. Keep your mind in the present and enjoy the experience. If you like running to music, create a killer playlist in the days leading up to the race. If you prefer the sounds of the forest, then take in the surroundings and get lost in the moment.

One technique to use is to look at an object in the near distance and run to it. Then pick another object a little farther and run to that. Then another, and another, and so on. This technique can help take your mind off the ultimate finish line. You can also focus on one aid station at a time. Let the goal be the next aid station. Celebrate each small victory and readjust your goals, keeping the finish line distant in your mind. Every small achievement will eventually be one amazing success.

Helpful Tip #9: Prevent Chafing

As a species, we've learned that friction creates fire – a discovery that changed the fate of humankind. But, when it comes to our bodies, not quite the discovery we want to feel in our running shorts! To prevent chafing, be sure to lube up in all friction spots. Furthermore, many runners choose to wear compression shorts to assist with sweat absorption. The two combined are a powerful combination in the fight against chafing.

Helpful Tip #10: Use This Priceless Energy

Race day is an incredible day with many mixed emotions. Nervousness is extremely common, especially if you're new to running or if it's your first ultramarathon. Bottle up that excitement and use it to your advantage. This type of energy is priceless – a type of energy you can't purchase online with a holiday promo code. I haven't run a single race that took more effort than what I accomplished in training. It's not the races that make us better as runners – it's the intense training and sacrifices we make to get us there. I look back at the time I ran ten ultra distances in preparation for my first 100-mile race. Or the mornings I walk out my door at 3:00 a.m. to run 30 miles in time to get home and feed my son's breakfast. Or the winter runs where my eyelids have literally frozen shut. The runs that don't end up with a finisher's buckle, tech shirt, and post-race meal. The type of runs with no official starting time, stocked aid stations, or results posted online. It's the type of run when you're only driven by the inspiration of the morning sun and the vision of achieving something incredibly distant in the unknown. So when you take that starting line, guess what? The hard work is done. The only thing left to do is stay focused, enjoy the ride, and run baby run!

Now that you have some help to get to the finish line, let's examine a critical aspect of the race. During your journey from start to finish, there is AID to help you along the way. What I'm referring to is 'aid stations,' and if you use them effectively, they can be of great AID. They can be the difference between a good and great day. So let's dive into aid stations and how to hit them effectively.

CHAPTER 9

Hit the AID Stations Right

The aid station is a short breath of fresh air from the punishing leg-pounding effects of an ultramarathon. It's a table of relief filled with volunteers, food, and drinks, and a few other odds and ends to aid you along the way. After running for hours along the same trail, sometimes it's just a relief to see another human being. Aid stations can be your best friend, and they can be your worst enemy. Become too comfortable too often, and you may fall victim to the lore of its temptations and never leave. So if you're new to ultrarunning listen up. Here are some of the most common questions answered about aid stations.

What exactly is an aid station?

An aid station is just that, a station with aid. It's typically made up of tables throughout an ultramarathon that supply aid to runners. Ultramarathons cover some extreme distances, so food and drinks are needed for fuel. Aid stations are stocked differently at each race, but they all have one common theme: aid.

What is supplied at an aid station?

Food, food, and ... did I say food? Aid stations have food, water, sports drinks, and energy gels. Some of the food you will find are potatoes, oranges, bananas, trail mix, candy, peanut butter and jelly sandwiches, salt, energy gels, almond butter, and sometimes even pizza. Some say jokingly that an ultramarathon is nothing more than an eating and drinking contest with a little exercise and scenery threw in. Also, you will likely find two or more fluid holders containing water and sports drinks. On hot days, you might see coolers of ice, while cold nights may include a fire or two. Other supplies sprinkle throughout the tables with sunblock, petroleum jelly, and first aid kits. Oh, and did I mention food?

How many aid stations are there during an ultramarathon?

Not enough! Well at least on race day, you will think so. Running those long endless miles may bring a lot of wishful thinking. Unfortunately, the wish never comes true. And every time you wish the next station was one mile closer, it feels two miles farther.

The number of aid stations per race will vary from a little to a lot. I ran an ultramarathon over 100 miles in length with nothing more than a few checkpoints and a cold bean quesadilla. But I ran an ultramarathon under 50 miles in length with an aid station every 4-5 miles containing a wide array of food. The point is this – the number of aid stations varies between races. If it's your first ultramarathon, try running one with an aid station located every 4-5 miles apart. A shorter distance between aid stations will also assist in staying on course and will help when the unexpected occurs.

Where can I find information on aid stations for my race?

Every ultramarathon I've ever seen had a website. On this site, you will find information on its aid stations. Also, as race day gets closer, the director will release informational emails on the event. Here you may find information on the aid stations, especially if they lack in numbers. If all else fails, be sure to send an email to the race director and ask your specific questions. No matter what people tell you, race directors are expecting a million and one questions, so just ask.

What if the aid stations do not stock my fuel of choice?

Well, what can I say? If ultramarathons were easy, everyone could do them. As ultrarunners, we are resourceful and if there's a will then there's a way. Sometimes an extremely long way, but still – a way.

Another answer is to use a drop bag. Most races will allow a drop bag where you can pack extra fuel and supplies. Also, determine if crew members are allowed at aid stations. This way, if you have specific fuel requirements, you may plan to meet your crew throughout the race. Finally, if all else fails, just put one foot in front of the other and keep moving forward. Eventually, by placing one foot in front of the other, you will reach the finish line, no matter what you eat.

Can my crew meet me at an aid station during the race?

Aid stations are usually found deep into the trails, and to access them from the outside is prohibited. Also, parking issues arise from the town's local authorities. Each race will have its own rules. I've run ultramarathons with one constant loop using one aid station. I've run a point-to-point with all different aid stations. I've even run an out-and-back hitting each aid station twice, and just about everything else. The point is to do your research, read the rules, and have a plan.

How long can you stay at an aid station?

It's such a relief to approach an aid station after a long stretch of what seems to be never-ending running. Reaching an aid station can be just what the doctor ordered to bring you back from the dead. They provide comfort, but too much comfort is harmful. There is no time limit at an aid station, but the key is efficiency. Personally, I grab whatever I need in a hurry and keep moving forward, adjusting and refueling on the move.

As you push through the sandstorms of each race day desert, the aid station is an oasis of relief. It sure puts your broken pieces back together when you need it most. It's there as your friend, but if you take advantage of it, then you may quickly become a victim of its seduction. So, get in, get out, and get moving along with what you set out to do. To run those miles, to keep moving forward, and to cross that finish line!

Now that you know how to hit the aid stations right, let's learn about the most effective ways to hydrate on race day.

CHAPTER 10

Water, Electrolytes, and a Little Technique

An effective hydration strategy is critical when running ultramarathon distances. There are various ways to go about it; however, what's most important is to choose a technique that works best for you. Our bodies are all different in how our electrolytes stay in balance on race day.

Here you will find a handful of techniques for hydrating when running an ultramarathon. So in your thirst for crossing the finish line of an ultramarathon, stay balanced, stay in control, and most importantly, stay hydrated.

The Super Hydrate Approach

Depending on your current hydration abilities, you may want to consider super hydrating. This technique requires a maximum intake of fluids at each aid station. The key is to hydrate to the maximum of your abilities until reaching the finish line. This technique is an empty-to-full approach because you flirt with the bare minimum of your hydration tank. If you choose to use this method, then it is best to bring along extra hydration gear. Also, be sure to hydrate in excess before the race begins. By hydrating your body above average before the race starts, you avoid any possibility of dehydration early on in the race.

The Weight Loss Approach

This systematic approach takes into account the amount of sweat lost per hour. To determine your sweat loss rate, weigh yourself naked before running. Next, run for one hour at race pace without sipping any fluids. If you must hydrate during your run, then record the number of ounces you drink. Lastly, after the completion of your run, wipe yourself entirely down of all sweat and weigh yourself naked again. Now you have your weight before your run, and after your run, this provides the difference in pounds. Convert the pounds to ounces and subtract any water intake. Your answer will provide the amount of water lost per hour. With this number, you will understand how much water you need for replenishment. Keep in mind: there are different variables which contribute to the outcome. For instance, perform this test in various weather conditions. Water loss through perspiration will vary in the cold versus in the heat. By completing this test in different weather, you will be ready for any adverse weather on race day.

The Time Interval Approach

Another hydration technique is to consume constant small sips throughout the entire race. For example, some people run with a hydration pack and take small sips throughout the race every 20 minutes. Most hydration packs hold up to 32 ounces of fluid, yet refill time is low. By using the time interval approach, running self-supported becomes easier. By holding more fluids and staying on a schedule, the dependence on aid stations reduces. On the flipside, a hydration pack creates more weight. Still, the time interval is a standard approach used by many ultramarathon runners.

The Drink When Thirsty Approach

This technique is the most simplistic approach. Run until you are thirsty, then re-hydrate. It is useful to bring along a hydration pack or a handheld bottle to assist you between aid stations.

So you may ask, "How do I know if I am dehydrated?" Typically, a runner knows when they are thirsty. Dry mouth, salty skin, or a slower pace can be dead giveaways. Also, you can monitor the color of your urine. Yes, the color of your urine. Look, ultrarunning is far from sexy, with little commercial appeal. Common race day practices like spilling drinks on yourself, urinating in bushes, and falling flat on your face have more in common with a 21st birthday party than a segment on ESPN. But we do whatever it takes to keep moving forward and to finish those long and exhausting miles. Those miles are self-demanding and can break you into pieces if you do not efficiently hydrate.

I cannot stress enough the importance of hydrating and of keeping your electrolytes in balance. It's essential to make good hydration habits a way of life, both in and out of your running shoes. Without proper hydration, your body cannot function properly. Then add in the level of stress an ultramarathon puts on your body, and it becomes even more difficult. Personally, I drink to thirst with water or coconut water. But there are a million and one different sports drinks to choose from that will help with hydration on race day. So, by using one of these techniques, you will be on your way to a smooth ultramarathon finish feeling energized, healthy, and fully hydrated.

Now that you have chosen a hydration approach, it's time to move on. Next, let's dive into the benefits of eating all natural and becoming fat adapted as an ultrarunner.

CHAPTER 11

Fat Is Your Friend

In today's competitive world of low-cost convenience, we have lost sight of the essential link between diet and physical activity. Take a car, for example. If you fill it with the correct gas and oil but fail to hit the pedal, then the car remains static. Eventually, it will lose battery power and rust away over time. On the other hand, if you put the pedal to the metal but put in the wrong gas and oil, then the car will break down. The same basic concept goes for exercise and running. If you eat healthily but train poorly then your goals become difficult to reach and may even cause injury. Conversely, if you train correctly but eat unhealthily, achieving your goals requires much more work. The two intertwine and the right combination leads to your ultimate success as a runner. It will lead to incredible outcomes, improved health, and an admirable physique. For ultrarunners, fat is your friend and an essential part of ultramarathon nutrition. It morphs you into a well-oiled machine and provides a nearly infinite supply of energy if metabolized efficiently. Yes, fat is your friend and here are the reasons why.

Fat, Sugar, and Calories

Did you know that on average, our bodies contain 160,000 calories and only roughly 5,000 are stored as sugar? So when you "hit the wall," the brain is shutting the muscles down to conserve sugar for the nervous system. The human's nervous system requires sugar to function. So if metabolized ineffectively, it leaves you up a creek without a paddle on race day. Fortunately, there are approximately 130,000 calories stored as fat in our bodies. So by training our metabolism to burn fat as its primary fuel source, energy becomes everlasting! Can you imagine the possibilities from this on race day?

Fight Or Flight and Sugar

Three words: fight or flight. What is fight or flight? It's a survival mechanism. As human beings, if we feel a threat to our survival, we can metabolize a whole lot of energy, and FAST. This vast amount of energy helps us cope with threats to our survival. Additionally, this quick rapid energy comes primarily from sugar. So let's relate this to running. If you are running fast, stopping, refueling with sports drinks and gels, running faster, and so on, then you are simulating a fight or flight pattern. You begin mimicking your ancestors. Those who were hunting and gathering for their survival for approximately... well, for the entire human existence. But, when you burn fat as your primary fuel source, your pace is much more moderate. This slow pace is far from a fight or flight state, causing you to refuel a lot less during an ultramarathon. Ultimately, this leads to longer miles and a more manageable experience.

Exercise and a Fat-Burning Metabolism

Want to become a fat-adapted ultramarathon runner? Well, it's certainly doable, but it takes time to achieve such a desirable change from within. I've been through it myself. While training, spend the majority of your time running in a comfortable aerobic state. A heart rate monitor works well to regulate this, but you can also figure this out without a heart rate monitor. If you can run at a pace where you can carry on a conversation, then you are running in a comfortable aerobic state. Personally, during my transitional training period, I felt sluggish, tired, and hungry. But I kept pushing farther and farther while moving faster and faster. I eventually pushed the limits to where I ran a 50k with no food or water. A zero intake for roughly 31 miles!

The key is to push past the concrete beliefs created by big business. Do this by ignoring the advertisements that persuade you to purchase unnecessary supplements. Once this occurs, you can listen to your body, and this is when the magic happens. Suddenly, you begin to crave the recipes provided by Mother Nature herself and live on your own terms! Then you have taken one giant leap towards becoming one sizable fat-burning machine.

Eat For Efficiency

Greens, greens, and more greens in addition to a habitual consumption of good fats like omega 3s. Eating this type of food is an adequate start towards an efficient fat burning metabolism. An ideal menu from a highly efficient fat burner is water, vegetables, nuts, salads, oils, vegetable soups, and fish. If this efficient fat burner consumed grains, than the grains would be low-starch. If eating greens through whole foods is difficult at first then try substituting with a green food powder. Preferably one labeled high in "alkalinity." These dietary health changes fight back against our hectic and acidic lifestyles. By making these changes it delivers life back into your body, creating energy through your entire day. Can you imagine the effects this will have on your running? Furthermore, it's just as important to keep sugar low during your runs as it is throughout your days. Although your body requires sugar during an ultramarathon, it's still possible to keep it at a minimal level. My fueling techniques are not perfect as I find myself consuming more fruits than I'd like. Personally, I just ran a 116-mile ultramarathon across the entire state of Florida. I fueled with water, coconut water, fruits, almonds, and vegetable broth and subsequently, finished in first place.

Sugar, Sugar, and More Sugar

As a society, we've become addicted to sugary processed substitutes. We label these alternatives as "food" and consume excessive amounts. Add in our limited sleep, overuse of caffeinated beverages, plus the pesticides and preservatives we consume through processed foods, and we put our bodies on one slippery slope to discomfort and disease. Next, from the effects of a poor diet, we are clinically diagnosed with disease and disorders. So we attempt to mask the symptoms with a magic pill when the root of the cause was never identified in the first place. We keep treating the effect instead of dealing with the cause. Only treating the symptoms encourages us to continue consuming an abundance of sugary processed foods. Moreover, as we take a ride on the blood sugar roller coaster, we rely more and more on sugar. But we hold each and every fat as the culprit. It's a vicious sugary cycle! If you understand this, then you can take corrective action and bring your running to new and healthy places.

When Enough Became Enough

After two years of ultrarunning, it seemed that every race led to an upset, nauseated stomach. I loved running ultramarathons, but things were getting worse. Every single race left me extremely nauseous towards the 25-30 mile mark. Nausea would intensify, haunting me for the rest of the race. I would then find myself curled up on the coach shortly after. I needed to figure this problem out and fast.

I began reading various articles in regards to how to eliminate nausea. There was advice like drinking soda or taking salt tabs, but I thought to myself, *why am I reading up on how to cure nausea?* That is, I was becoming nauseated for a reason. A better question would be, *why do I become nauseous? And how do I prevent it from happening?* There had to be a reason why my body became ill every time I raced. I rejected the notion that it was from running such long mileage. I believe we as human beings have accomplished only a fraction of our actual capabilities.

So after trial and error and some pattern recognition, I took a chance. I decided to eliminate all processed foods from my diet. Making these changes naturally reduced my sugar intake in the process. I eliminated these foods both during races and between races. I began changing my entire lifestyle, and you know what? I cured my stomach issues immediately. In addition, if nausea did arise on race day, I would then drastically reduce my sugar intake. The elimination of processed foods and sugary fuel was the cure-all.

It's amazing how sometimes the answers are right in front of us. Since the norm was sugary sports drinks and gels, I was programmed to only accept this as a fueling option. But ultramarathons are not normal. So why should I have been fueling normally? Between the countless gels, energy blocks, and sugary sports drinks, not to mention the number of carbohydrates I was eating within a 24 hour period, it was no wonder that my stomach hurt. Better yet, with these fueling habits, nausea was a near guarantee. It was a sugary, explosive massacre of a diet, and my stomach was the victim.

Shortly after, my perception changed dramatically on eating and dieting. Our food grows in a natural form so why shouldn't you eat it in a natural form? Furthermore, diets began to make little to no sense to me. Why would you "diet" when you are not eating naturally to begin with? If you always eat your food in a natural state, then no special diet is ever needed. It's not a diet change but a lifestyle change that's necessary. Change the way you eat and change your life forever.

Man had three evolutionary discoveries that changed how we would live our lives forever. Fire, the wheel, and... the drive-thru window. Yes, the drive-thru window. Over time, this convenience has contributed to our explosively high sugary and acidic lifestyles. What it's done is create convenience in place of consciousness. But if you can take advantage of our potential energy – that is, the fat already stored within our bodies, you can then have a nearly infinite supply of energy. Slow and steady like a coal fire burning, you can move forward through a new way of training that will not only change the way that you run, but it will also change the way that you live your life. Remember, even with the greatest diet on earth, those miles will never run themselves. There is no magic formula besides putting in those long miles and moving forward. But, along those paths less traveled, it's beneficial to pick up a friend or two along the way. For ultrarunners, fat is your friend and one you can certainly depend on.

Now, let's shift entirely from fueling and nutrition. Let's dive into what I like to call "mounds of opportunity."

CHAPTER 12

Hills = Mounds of Opportunity

How a runner handles the uphill battle determines what they're made of. That's in ultrarunning and life as well. How do you achieve growth the quickest? Well, that depends on the amount of resistance a runner is willing to take. Fortunately for runners, hills are resistance in its rawest form. During an ultramarathon, a runner could face anywhere between 30 to 30,000 feet of elevation gain. Sometimes even higher! With this in mind, strategizing your hill climbs is essential. Love them or hate them, like it or not, elevation gain is an everyday commonality for an ultrarunner. So to help, here's some typical hill running techniques for ultramarathons.

Technique #1: Train For Them

First things first, let's keep things simple. The key to hill training is training on the same elevation that you will face on race day. So where do you find different elevation? Well, the beauty of the outdoors is also its hidden benefit – that is, no one thing is the same. You'll never see two of the same rocks, trees, paths, etc. One trail can be long and flat while the other can be short and steep. So find a trail or road that matches your race day elevation. No elevation where you live? Well then, become familiar with treadmill inclines, StairMasters, and parking garages.

One time when I hurt my knee, I trained solely on a

StairMaster for an upcoming race. I increased my mileage incrementally, eventually reaching one workout of 37 miles. I walked up those spinning steps for six whole hours, never once touching the sidebars. There was indeed a lot of time spent staring at the gym wall, building exceptional mental strength. I also used an iPad to watch movies, along with an endless playlist of new music.

The take-home here is this: be more creative than your excuses and train on inclines similar to what you'll see on race day.

Technique #2: Small Quick Steps

As I stressed in a previous chapter, keep your strides small and quick uphill. This will change the overall dynamic of a runner's motion. Try this: first, while progressing uphill, take a few lunges. Next, make your way up the same hill, but this time, take small shorter steps. Which takes less effort? It's the latter every time. Similar to shifting a bike to a lower gear, a shorter step requires more revolutions but less energy per revolution. The change in motion can feel as if you're running on flat terrain. In this way, the hills begin to disappear, and your experience becomes much more enjoyable on race day.

Technique #3: Speed Hike

Another technique for race day is to walk the hills. Place your hands on your hips or knees, or swing those arms and speed hike upwards. Once on top, begin running, and make up your time on the downhills. Fly down those quad-screaming descents with the brakes released, and watch gravity work its magic.

Ever lose too much energy during a race? If you look at your race day energy as a bank, walking hills provides an evenly distributed withdraw on race day. This way you reach the finish line before going broke.

Technique #4: Run Them, Run Them Fast

Run those hills and take the beating! Running hills full out is the most basic technique of the bunch. Sure, this may not be the most strategic, but sometimes you just do what you have to do. Here's the trick: once you reach the top, and run entirely through the hill, slow your pace down. From here wait until you're re-energized, and pick it right back up to a race-day pace.

Technique #5: Use Trekking Poles

Some ultramarathons have such demanding vertical gains that they allow trekking poles. But here's the catch, once you decide using them, you must hold them for the entire race. No ditching them off at the next aid station – that extra weight is yours to the finish. They become your friend until the end!

Technique #6: Embrace The Hills

Hills: the good, the bad, and the extremely painful. Hills will always be present. One way or another, they are always waiting, patiently and persistently. So, find the hill first, or the hill will find you! Personally, I've learned to embrace the hills during ultramarathons. They are a change of pace, a break for other muscles, and a chance to see some pretty unbelievable views. So don't worry, once you decide to embrace the hills then you will be in luck! You will be in luck because once you reach the top of one hill, there is always another hill to follow.

Ultramarathons can be challenging, and the hills can be the toughest part. I remember some races where I felt like my shoes transformed into cement blocks! It felt like I couldn't run another inch, let alone another 50 miles. But I also remember some hills that made me stronger and brought me a front row ticket to some of the most magnificent views I've ever seen.

Hills will always be available, but they are only relative to the resistance you're adapted to. I've seen flatlanders drop out of hilly races, and interestingly enough, I've seen skyrunners drop out of flat races. Either way, if you choose a technique and push against the resistance of the hill, your body will adapt. Hills will transform you into a stronger and faster ultrarunner. An ultrarunner who can run up those hills instead of away from them!

Yes, I did say some ultrarunners do drop out. Unfortunately, it happens during every race. Many factors contribute to this. Fortunately, I have not dropped out of a race yet, so I will provide tips to help avoid dropping out yourself. Next, let's discuss some of the most common reasons for dropping out. Avoiding these mistakes will help you avoid a DNF, meaning: "did not finish."

CHAPTER 13

Don't Quit! #DNF

The dreaded three letters in ultrarunning: DNF or Did Not Finish. The three letters that no ultrarunner at any level wants to hear on race day. Ultramarathons are different from any other endurance event. While running an ultramarathon, you can only expect this: expect the unexpected. Things will go wrong, and things will go right. There are many highs and many lows during an ultramarathon, but there is some good news. That is, if you keep moving forward and avoid some common mistakes, the finish line is entirely achievable. To help you reach the finish on race day, here are some of the most common mistakes that lead to a DNF.

Starting Too Fast = DNF

As I explained earlier when the race begins, it's common to get a rush of adrenaline, and you may not even realize it. When this happens, if you are new to ultrarunning, you tend to run too fast too soon and end up burning out. Its a long day, and burning out too early will lead to exhaustion and possibly a DNF.

One 100-mile ultramarathon I ran consisted of 4 out-and-backs that were 25 miles each in length. After the first 25 miles, I felt burnt out. The heat index reached 110 degrees Fahrenheit, and I did not compensate for such extreme heat. After completing 50 miles, I could not comprehend nor could I rationalize running another 50 miles to the finish. It's a lonely place to be exhausted 50 miles into a 100-mile race. However, what I did was simple, I kept my mind in the present and continued moving my feet forward. At times it seems like a race will never come to an end, but one way or another, it does. So in the moment, as runners, you can do what you do best, and that is, keep moving your feet forward and run!

Sitting Down = DNF

In ultrarunning there is a saying: "Beware of the chair!" On race day, it's a good idea always to move forward and refrain from sitting down if you can avoid it. Walk if you must. When you stop moving during an ultramarathon, you become weak, stiff, and tired. Starting back up takes a substantial amount of energy. Avoiding the chair will help prevent muscle fatigue and a DNF on race day.

The temperature during my first 100-mile ultramarathon exceeded 80 degrees during the day. After some evening thunderstorms, the temperatures plummeted down to the 40s. I will never forget my first encounter with the mantra "beware of the chair." When I ran up to an aid station late into the night, a runner was wrapped up in a blanket, shivering next to a fire. Apparently, when he took a seat at the aid station, his body went into a mild shock, forcing him to remain in the chair until deciding on his DNF. In the cold, especially when the sun is down, try to continue moving. If you must walk then pump your arms forcefully and rapidly, then get back to running when you can. Just never stop moving forward and most importantly, beware of the chair!

Experimenting With New Fuel = DNF

Using only gel may be adequate for marathon distances but not so much in ultramarathon distances. If you attempt to use the same gel for, say, 100 miles, you may quickly find yourself for the majority of the race trying not to throw up on your shoes. Try to practice eating whole foods during your training runs. Trial and error is essential during training. It will help you find new fuel sources, avoiding experimentation on race day that could lead to nausea and vomiting. If nausea is unavoidable, try ginger chews or chicken broth to help settle your stomach.

Here's another lesson I learned from my first 100-mile ultramarathon. As I mentioned in a prior chapter, I fueled with a gel for 50 miles until my stomach began to reject it. By using solely gels, I became extremely nauseous. During the entire remaining 50 miles, I was immeasurably nauseous. It took everything in me to not throw up. I began fueling with a water bottle filled with chicken broth and water. I forced down just about anything to keep my caloric intake somewhat above par. It was a devastating feeling; however, I blocked nausea out of my mind and somehow held it together to the finish.

From that day forward, I swore off all sugary gels and sports drinks and began to eat only whole foods. Processed foods have been eliminated from my life for quite some time now. It quickly turned into one of the best decisions of my life as it provided me an entirely different outlook on nutrition. Those who fuel naturally will understand. It's a nutritional opportunity that sits right in front of all of us. Your body feels incredible when you choose whole foods over quick pops of sugary processed substitutions. It could change your running journey in unbelievable ways. Looking back at that day, I realized it was a blessing in disguise. Sometimes you must become extremely disturbed to make a change in your life. Don't get me wrong, I always ate what I thought to be healthy, but from this experience, I learned what healthy truly is. So would I have made such a radical shift in my eating habits if this nutritional catastrophe had not occurred? Possibly, but I would not have taken action as quickly nor be as consistent in the dietary changes I've made. It's not what we do every so often that creates change that is lasting; instead, it's what we do consistently.

Not Applying Anti-Chafing Lube = DNF

Lube up in all friction spots with a petroleum-based product. You will thank yourself later in the race. Reapply during the race periodically and proactively–more so if it is raining. Compression gear can also help. Chafing can be a big issue during ultramarathons if you are not prepared. During more extended events, consider changing your clothes periodically. Chafing is a common reason for a DNF. If all else fails, throw on some duct tape and keep your legs moving forward to the finish.

During that same 100-mile ultramarathon that consisted of 4 out-and-backs, the last 25 miles were the toughest. It wasn't tough because of the lack of sleep, nausea, or fatigue. The day of running in the sun and rain came back to haunt me. It was the toughest because of the intense chafing I was experiencing. The chafing got so painful that it felt like razor blades were rubbing against me with each step. The pain was unbearable. When I reached the aid station at the turn around it was time to get creative and resourceful. I grabbed two shirts, a roll of duct tape, a bottle of Vaseline, and a bag of cornstarch. I duct taped one shirt under my shorts and poured down half the bag of cornstarch. The cornstarch was an incredible alternative to baby powder. I put on the other shirt, lifting the front behind my head, so it propped my arms, up preventing them from rubbing against my underarms. Here I applied some vaseline and cornstarch. This jiffy lube of ultrarunning plus the Sunday morning sunrise gave me some life back as I pushed myself across the finish line.

Taking Too Much Time at Aid Stations = DNF

Keep your eye on the clock. If you take too much time at aid stations, you could find yourself flirting with the cutoff times. Missing a cutoff time is another common reason for a DNF. As you run up to an aid station, have your mental checklist ready, grab what you need, and walk forward as you organize your fuel. Once you're ready, get right back to running.

Personally, I do not run into an issue with cutoff times; however, I'd like to give kudos to those runners who take the max time to finish an ultramarathon. When the aid stations are closing down, and the race is coming to an end, some runners are still out there running. They move relentlessly to the finish, sometimes even past cutoff times. That's drive, that's motivation, that's sheer mental strength, and I congratulate you for it.

Water/Electrolyte Imbalance = DNF

It's essential to manage the balance between your water intake and your electrolytes (sodium, potassium, calcium, etc.) When your electrolytes are out of balance, it can lead to cramping and a DNF. Be sure to monitor your water and salt intake. Runners use salt tablets, electrolyte powder, chicken broth, salted potatoes, and sports drinks. You can also monitor your hydration by the color and frequency of your urine output. An electrolyte imbalance can be dangerous, so be careful. Be sure to make safe choices on race day and cross that finish line hydrated and healthy.

During a 50k, I did not do a great job keeping my electrolytes balanced and was running well above my 50k race day pace. Suddenly and without warning, I cramped up intensely. I immediately grabbed my leg and fell to the ground. My hamstrings tightened up as I arched my back, performing one of those laughing yells. You know, when it hurts so you yell but laugh because you know how funny you look. I was squirming on the ground in the middle of the woods with no one in sight. I think even a deer shook its head at me and kept on its way. To adjust, I took baby strides to the next aid station and super-hydrated upon arrival. Fortunately, I bounced back and finished with no other problems.

Ignoring Minor Irritations = DNF

Small irritations can evolve into painful circumstances on race day. A pebble in your shoe at the beginning of a race can eventually feel like a boulder towards the end of a race. This also goes for rubbing, blisters, and sunburn. If you feel hotspots on your feet or experience foot pain, try to re-tie your shoes or change them at the aid station. Blisters are one of the top reasons for a DNF, so be proactive and prevent them early on.

In ultramarathons, we find this mistake to be most accurate. It's a smart idea to stay in-tune with how your body feels.

There have been times where a small pebble has actually put a hole in my big toe. So don't ignore the minor irritations.

Many factors can contribute to receiving a DNF on race day. But when managed effectively, you can avoid them with no problem. Besides handling the physical issues, you also must give importance to the mental aspect of the race. Staying in the right place mentally on race day, in my opinion, is the most crucial aspect of all. So next, let's dive into the mental aspect of running ultramarathons. Let's apply mind over matter.

CHAPTER 14

Mind Over Matter

Yes, you run the first 50 miles of an ultramarathon with your body and the second 50 miles with your mind. I say this from experience. When the pain in your legs is unbearable, and the chafing on your body is torturous, it's mental strength that will carry you through to the finish. I've run for 60 miles, and it's felt like bliss, and conversely, I've run 30 miles, and it's felt like misery. The power of your mental stamina dictates which of the two experiences you will go through.

So, as help on the big day, here you will find some mental strategies that will help you complete an ultramarathon. Your mind is your greatest strength! Your mind is the key to unlock greatness within yourself to run ultramarathon distances.

Mental Strategy #1: Stay in the Present

Training your mind to stay in the present is sometimes challenging. Focusing on a finish line or the end of a race is a natural tendency for most runners. We pound and pound through an intense amount of stress, only to reach the ultimate relief from the finish. But what if you could find relief within your run? That's what staying in the present accomplishes. It allows you to become aware of the moment. There are many techniques; however, morning meditation is the most common. Our mental muscles strengthen with morning meditation, and it transitions well into running.

Mental Strategy #2: Find an Object

When running such long and taxing distances, the mental challenges become the most difficult to overcome. Can you imagine having 99 miles to go in any type of race, let alone one completed by running? Comprehending such a challenge is tough. At times, you can become stuck in a mental rut, fixated on the finish line, causing you to lose focus on the present. One mental technique to help shift your attention back to the "now" is finding an object in the distance and running to it. Then, find one further and run to that. Then, further, and further, and so on, until you find your groove again. By reaching each new checkpoint, it will provide a small victory. This small victory will help remove the focus away from the finish line back to the present.

Mental Strategy #3: Break It Up

An ultramarathon can be overwhelming at times. Reasons to quit are always available, but, good news: so are reasons to finish. To help minimize the overwhelmedness of an ultramarathon, try to break the race up by aid station. In this way, the race will only be as far as the next aid station ahead, nothing shorter and nothing longer. By using this strategy, each small achievement will eventually grow into one GIANT success.

Isn't this true for any of your dreams in life? What's most important is each small achievement; the small actions you take each day towards your goals. When you set big goals and take action, it shapes you into the person who is capable of achieving them. Ever notice after every race that within a week or so, you begin choosing your next challenge? After every run, I think to myself "Never again!" Until the next day when I find myself thinking "What's next!?"

Mental Strategy #4: Make A List

"Why am I doing this?" "What's the point?" "Who in their right mind would do this to themselves?" These are just a few of the questions one may ask while running deep into the painful moments of an ultramarathon. There will be ups and there will be downs, so be proactive. Try this: create a small list of reasons in which you decided to take on such a challenge in the first place. Naturally, you will try to talk yourself out of finishing; it's fight or flight at its finest. I can't tell you how many excuses I've blocked out during the many ultra distances I've run thus far. But remember, an excuse is just that: an excuse. How you feel from a particular experience is only determined by the meaning you give it. With a list of your "whys," it will provide the kryptonite to slay those air-filled excuses. You can then keep moving forward down the trails to the finish line in a positive state of mind.

Mental Strategy #5: Know Your Mantra

Create an inspiring and purpose-driven mantra or find a quote that sincerely moves you. When times get tough on the course – and trust me, times will get tough – begin repeating that mantra. Repeat it in your mind or say it out loud, over and over again. Repeating your mantra is a great way to pull you out from those race day lows.

Or better yet, add a song to your playlist that truly inspires you. You know, that song that gives you the chills every time you hear it. Once you've decided on the song, create a new playlist. Next, add the song 20 times. This way, when you slip into a low point on the race, that unavoidable valley, turn on

the song and play it over and over again until you're back upon a peak. Sing if it helps! Running with high spirits can provide an incredible experience on ultramarathon race day.
The idea is to find your mantra or a song that's close to your heart. Then bring it out when the going gets tough, because as an ultramarathon runner, the tough get going. Like your physical strength, your mental strength needs a constant workout to develop and grow. Positive mantras and inspiring songs will help you continue to run when you can't. When you push past your comfort zone, this is when you experience growth!

Mental Strategy #6: Next Day Blues

As the pain sets in and the doubts take a chop at your legs, to help, try visualizing the following day. Sometimes it feels like a race will never end, but they always do. Regardless of the outcome, one way or another, tomorrow always comes. The only difference will be how much of yourself was left on the course. Therefore, if you think back on the day, and you gave every ounce possible, there will be zero regrets. In life, you get to choose: the pain of discipline or the pain of regret. And guess what? The pain of discipline weighs mere ounces, compared to the pain of regret, and it will only make you better. So at that moment when you feel weak, then find the strength! When you feel tired, then find the energy! When you feel doubtful, then find the courage! Courage is not when you know you can achieve a goal; it's when you're unsure or afraid and you push forward anyway. It is when you have faith in yourself and faith in the unknown. So that next day, when you're sitting and reflecting on the race, the pain in your legs will feel a little better. Because if you have given your all, you can smile and lay down with zero regrets. You just ran an ultramarathon and can now reflect on your extraordinary race day performance.

Mental Strategy #7: Lose the Watch

A few years ago, I was traveling towards the beach for a summer vacation on the east coast of the United States. On the car ride there, I jumped out 37 miles from my destination. At the time, this was my longest attempted distance for a training run. Ultrarunning was still new to me, and everything was going well until around the 28th mile. All of a sudden, I began to lose it! My eyes became glued to my watch and every minute seemed like an eternity until I 'eventually started to walk. It now reminds me of the time I rode 100 miles on a stationary bike or when I spent 6 hours on a StairMaster, a slave to the digital countdown of time. Enough was enough. I took off the GPS watch attached to my wrist and launched it as far as my arm could throw it. You see, I learned something about myself that day. That day, I learned that monitoring my time, splits, and pace while running did not motivate me – actually, it did the exact opposite. For me, checking my pace over and over again added an extra weight on my shoulders. Monitoring my running through a watch beat me down mentally. Losing the watch helps me keep my mind in the present and to continue moving forward on race day. I lose track of how far I've headed and how far I have left, so I just run. Ultimately, there's never been a finish line but a continuous journey to travel.

Mental Strategy #8: Know the Why

To have a mileage goal is excellent. But taking action to reach that goal is really what it's all about. There's power in the process. So before reaching the starting line, know your "why." Why do you want to take on such a challenge and why is it so important? Personally, what inspires me most about ultrarunning is unknown mysteries. For myself, ultrarunning has been a way that a 9 to 5 working athletic dad has the opportunity to "walk on the moon." Running a new mileage like 100 miles takes your physical, mental, and spiritual self into the unknown – and you don't need a pair of moon boots to get you there.

Mental Strategy #9: Talk With Fellow Runners

Chatting with your fellow competitors while running will help pass the time. At some point or another, it's fair to say every runner enjoys at least a few words during a race – some more than others – but a few reassuring words will always be beneficial. Personally, I've always admired people for their differences. So although I prefer running alone, not even using a pacer, I've met some incredible people on the trails. During an ultramarathon, we all have an understanding to some degree of what each other is going through. We can all relate on some painful level.

Mental Strategy #10: Bring Your Support System

Family and friends welcome. For some, having support on race day can be just the boost a runner needs to keep those legs moving forward. Just seeing a familiar face after running hours alone in the woods can be a relief. I've carried my sons across many finish lines, moments that I will never forget.

Mental Strategy #11: Race Against Yourself

For most, the real race is the one against yourself. Create a mental edge by focusing on the overall mileage or time. Push yourself to beat that real opponent, that voice deep down that screams to stop. That's the true competition, the one from within.

Mental Strategy #12: Be Competitive

Racing against another runner can be motivating. Motivation through competition is a great way increase your efforts. Mostly, ultramarathons are a race against yourself, but sometimes you find a match. If you're a top contender that day, then racing for the top spot can keep your body pushing for that first place finish. I've been there, and it's funny how even after 100 miles it always comes down to the wire. It's almost as if the previous 90 plus miles becomes irrelevant and it's a new race. The new race becomes those last few miles, and you're pushing through them with an empty tank.

During an ultramarathon, it's essential to keep moving your feet forward despite the struggle. If you relentlessly move forward when the body gives up, suddenly your mental strength becomes the driving force. When this occurs, the mind and the body are no longer in harmony working together. They have become two separate entities fighting for dominance. The body is wanting to quit while the mind is wanting to continue. This contradiction is "that place" or "that moment" which very few people outside the world of endurance sports have experienced. By choosing to self-impose such physical pain as opposed to having an outside event cause the pain is puzzling. Like when you ask someone why they climbed a mountain, and they reply, "Because it was there."

It is in "that place" or "that moment" of every extreme situation where all the cliches of triumph and victories are born. To most people, it may seem like just a race. But to endurance athletes, it is a self-defining moment. Your mind has won over your incredibly conditioned but exhausted body. Finishing an ultramarathon happens from the chin up, it's mind over matter. If your head doesn't mind, then your body doesn't matter.

Next, on the subject of mental strength, let's dive into some help in staying motivated. In the next chapter, you will learn how to stay motivated as an ultrarunner.

CHAPTER 15

Staying Motivated

Once your first ultramarathon is complete, the question becomes: how do you stay motivated? That is, how do you continue training and racing at such enduring distances? The key is in your mindset and how you can increase your motivation over time.

Time is always changing, and as a runner, you continuously move towards something. Your movement can be forwards or backward but either way, you are forever changing.

We are dynamic creatures by nature. But sometimes moving forward through your training program can become difficult. Backing off your mileage is more comfortable and a lot easier. But as runners, we all need to grow and progress. This is what steers us to become runners in the first place.

So, as an ultrarunner, how do you move forward through your training program to each new starting line? Well, the foundation begins with MOTIVATION and here are some tricks to help.

Variety Equals Growth

When you are stuck, bored, or tired, try to interrupt the pattern. To break up these habits, do something completely unexpected. When you add variety and intensity to your runs, it puts new demands on your body and keeps running fresh in your mind. For example, during long runs, you can sprint full speed every 15 minutes for 1 minute. Run as if you were breaking your record for a quarter-mile time.

Another technique is adding more hills to your run. By running more hills, you will force your body to raise its heart rate while training. In turn, the body increases its aerobic and anaerobic capacities in the process. So, in the end, you improve your stamina, power, speed, and overall strength. You see, hills create more variety and intensity. When you add them to your training runs, you come to realize this is exactly what's required to make a change. Variety and intensity are precisely what you need to progress and snap out of your same old running routine. It's what allows you to avoid and break free of running plateaus, both physically and mentally.

Cross training also adds variety to your running. Not just that, but it takes you out of your comfort zone, which is the key to growth. Isn't it true that stepping outside your comfort zone is how you ultimately become better at anything? Years ago I felt uncomfortable running outside for the first time, and now I never run on a treadmill. Remember, every time you step outside your comfort zone, growth is guaranteed. We all need some variety in our lives, so be creative, and keep your body on its toes – literally.

Set Your Goals With the Outcome in Mind

Be sure to have your next race picked out before beginning a new training session. Training for an ultramarathon with a race deadline is useful. Did you ever notice how you perform with a deadline versus without one? Aren't you much more productive with one? Remember, a goal is nothing more than a dream with a deadline.

You can also consider what meeting that deadline means to you. Remember a time you overcame a difficult challenge and achieved your goal? How did that make you feel? There is much more reward for completing your training than relief from quitting halfway through. When you attempt and reach your goals, it provides you with genuine happiness. But, if you're not achieving your desired goals, then you may want to consider changing your approach. For instance, if your knee hurts, then consider reevaluating your approach. Try changing your training schedule, technique, or shoes. The decisions we make and the goals that we set are what make us take action in running; they are what shape the future of our sport.

While running one day, I saw a bird in the sky, flying as a morning storm set in and the wind picked up intensely. The bird was flapping its wings with all its might, but unfortunately, it was not moving anywhere. Waving and flapping, over and over again, but staying in the same place. No matter how much effort the bird gave, it could not fly forward. It even began to move backward at one point. After trying and trying, failing and failing, over and over again, can you guess what happened? The bird decided to change its approach. It straightened its wings, becoming aerodynamic and instantly zipped forward. The bird went from a struggle going nowhere to eventually soaring effortlessly into the wind. Sometimes while running, you may use too much force and believe more running will solve all issues. But if you take a step back and adjust your approach, then you can run and progress with far less work. Running will suddenly become more enjoyable, bringing you to more starting lines. Learning how to improve with less effort will provide you with longevity in the sport.

Sign Up for the Race

I remember signing up for my first regular marathon years ago. It took a lot of courage. I remember the hesitation I experienced just to put my name on the list. At the time, my longest run was 14 miles in length. Before I signed up, I went to a nearby track and ran 20 miles. Wow, do I remember how my legs hurt afterward! When I signed up for my first ultramarathon, I had plenty of doubts. When I think back, there was no real level of comfort before signing up. I just ripped the Band-Aid off, entered my name, and decided on race day I'd just move forward and hold on for dear life. Signing up for a race sets your goal in concrete. It makes it real in your mind, and you then turn your thoughts into things, real things. Now that your goal is real, you will begin to do what's necessary to reach the starting line.

Leverage Your Motivation

Find out what motivates you and use it to your advantage. Love new clothes? Buy a new running outfit. Does time motivate you? Increase your pace. Are you a social butterfly? Run with other people. My prime time for running is early in the morning – that is, when I feel and move in an effortless motion. If I feel stuck in a rut during a morning run, I'll then run a late night long run. That way, my next morning long run feels fresh, and I move much faster. For example, for my last one-hundred-mile race, I ran a 33-mile training run in the morning but felt heavy. My head felt entirely out of it. So the next week, I ran a 37-miler through the night. It was tiring, very tiring, and oh yeah, did I mention I was tired? Not to mention I couldn't find an open store anywhere. After miles with no luck, I found myself standing in the movie theatre line shirtless to buy a bottle of water. Anyway, the next weekend I ran a 42-mile training run in the morning and felt explosive! This time around I felt refreshed and light compared to my Saturday night movie run. Sometimes, things need to become a little worse before they become better again, and they always become better with time.

Motivation is Everywhere

If you look, there is motivation everywhere. Our world is flooded with motivational tales of individuals taking on astounding challenges. Some swim across oceans, and some run across deserts. There are movies about space explorations, athletic achievements, and fighting racial oppression. There are readings from activists, poets, and philosophers that inspire us all. The point is when you see what's possible from others, your challenges become realistic. Get moving out of the door and towards your next starting line when you become INSPIRED.

A few years back, I was watching ESPN while they were headlining a woman who swam across the Atlantic Ocean. At the time, I was not training for anything in particular. After watching this woman's interview, I was instantly inspired. She spoke with a worn body and swollen face; it was just incredible. So, that day after work, I went home and spontaneously ran 31 miles. It was sparked solely by the inspiration I developed that day. Inspiration is contagious in your quest to do great things in your lives. So, keep your ears and eyes open for anything that will inspire you during training. Run your next training run with a newfound energy, natural energy, energy you created from within.

Skip a Training Run

If you miss a training run, it doesn't mean you've failed and must stop. Ask any seasoned ultrarunner, and I'm sure they've missed a training run in the past and still continued to race day. Whenever you miss a training run, move onto the next one; just don't make it a habit. Over and over again, I see people want to run their first standard marathon but give up on their training. The problem is that they pick a training schedule where they run 5-6 days a week and burn out. They think the more they run, the better. But running 5-6 days a week as a beginner will most likely lead to exhaustion or injury. These are the most common causes of missed training runs leading to a failed attempt. The goal of my first ultramarathon was to get across the finish line, and my training reflected that.

Be Conscious of the Benefits

I know, running an ultramarathon isn't always the healthiest form of physical activity. Nevertheless, here's what I will tell you from personal experience. The lifestyle changes I've made to be able to endure these distances have been incredible. Ultrarunning has changed my life for the better. The benefits have far outweighed the harm of what any distance could do. For example, eating all natural, not drinking alcohol or going out late. Plus, avoiding everything that tags along with my old bad habits and poor choices. The benefits of ultramarathon running have affected me in such an incredible way that it's hard to put into words. Not to mention the reduction in stress or how you deal with it. To do what you love alone can change your life forever. So focus on the benefits, monitor your progress, and acknowledge your outcomes. Every day is a good day when you run.

The Power of Music and Friends

Before every new long run, I try to download a new playlist. I regularly find new songs when I'm out, search them on my phone, and then I screenshot the results to download later. I've done this in department stores, in the car, and while watching movies. Music is a great way to empower your run, sort of like running with a group; it provides more power and determination. Have you ever noticed the first thing you want to do when something exciting happens in your life? Immediately, you want to share it with someone. Sharing your experiences helps you experience them again. Running with people can add the same type of benefit. Music and friends can provide exceptional motivation. The kind of motivation that gets those legs through your next training program.

Growing up, I did not listen to country music. Never had an interest in it and never thought I would. One day at work, I was on the phone sitting on hold, listening to a song playing on the other end of the phone. I searched the lyrics online, and it was a new country song. Not thinking anything of it, I added the song to my playlist for my first upcoming 100k. Well, on race day the song came on while I was at a peak state of mind. The song went on repeat, and it stayed on a repetitive loop for the next 30 miles straight! Since then, country music has filled my playlist, along with many other genres. It's no longer about the type of music; it's now about the song that moves my soul. Music is energy, music is fuel, and yes, music is motivation.

Gain Mental Strength

Your mental strength builds in congruence with your physical strength. This relationship is especially true in ultramarathon running. As I stressed earlier, make your training program only as long as your next run. Can't imagine running 50 miles? Don't. Imagine running 5 miles, then imagine running 10 miles, then imagine running 20 miles, and so on. Think about it: if you're new to weight lifting and attempt to bench press 300lbs, you will be in trouble. Chances are you'd quickly find yourself trapped under the bar. It works in both directions. Your psychological strength will build just as your physical strength will build. In the ultra-world, your mental strength is most important and this is an advantage. Think about it; your physical muscles are only really working out as long as you run. But your mental strength never shuts off. Our minds are working 24/7 even when we are sleeping. So be sure to sharpen your mental strength through visualization. For example, crossing the finish line of your first ultramarathon. Here's a thought – close your eyes if you must – how do you feel when you HOPE to finish a race? Now, how do you feel when you EXPECT to finish a race? Feel the difference? What you achieve governs what you believe, your potential is limitless!

A Boost from the Sun

Would you like an extra boost of energy while running? Try using the sunrise for motivation. Get out on your run while it's still dark and catch that sunrise bright and early. It shifts your internal clock forward as your body realizes the new day has come. When running 24 hours into the next morning, you experience this phenomenon. One time during an ultramarathon, I fell asleep while running! Ultramarathons

CHAPTER 15: Staying Motivated

that extend through the night are tiring, but when sunrise takes place, you feel alive again. Your body is now aware of the new day, and the boost of energy received is powerful. The sunrise is motivational, it's inspirational, and it's energizing. The morning sun gives you just enough energy to drive yourself forward to the completion of your run.

As endurance athletes, we are always in search of something more significant. And as people and as athletes, are we in the search for something more? Of course we are. As a species, we went from spending our days in the wild fighting for our survival to spending our days in a square home eating a boxed lunch.

By running and pushing myself, I can only hope it inspires others to move further in their own running. I hope you become inspired the same way I was a few years ago when I first got into distance running. It wasn't from someone running behind me screaming, "You can do it!" In this, you might obtain motivation but would never sustain it. No, it was the inspiration that naturally grew inside me. It grew from watching a man I know push past inconceivable levels of health and fitness. From there, I became inspired, and I kept the momentum alive, and it still is. I've continued well past what I ever could have possibly fathomed. And you know what the best part is? If you choose to keep growing, then you are only at the start of your journey. Motivation is what keeps you moving, but the key to long-term motivation is INSPIRATION. You will soon learn inspiration is contagious, and in that sense, I hope you caught some from this chapter!

Now that you can stay motivated as an ultramarathon runner, let's discuss what makes a successful one. Next, I will lay out the three secret ingredients to a successful ultramarathon runner.

CHAPTER 16

The Secret Ingredients

Through the many ultramarathons I've run, I've accumulated a lot of hands-on endurance experience. Not only in regards to achieving rapid growth, but to focusing on longevity and long-term health as well. Recently I read a quote that said, "If a coach can't do it, they cannot 'teach' it, only 'talk' about it." Whether that's true or not, I can confidently say that I write from experience. When spending so much time on long runs, you begin to notice patterns. For example, patterns of what is beneficial, not just for your next race but your long-term strategy as well. Yes, as runners, you must all do what works best for yourself. But I believe there are also three universal ingredients to a successful ultrarunner, and here they are.

Secret Ingredient #1: Focus

Decisions, decisions, decisions. We must be 100% certain and committed to the race of our choosing. When you sign up for a race, you must be 100% committed. If you want to achieve it, then you must believe it. Believe that it's possible, believe in your training, and believe in the outcome. Three words that sum it up are "GO ALL IN." If the new distance excites you: great, let the possibility of pleasure motivate you. If you're afraid of failing: even better, let the thought of pain bring out your determination from inside. Think about it: can you remember a time when you've given intense focus to an outcome? Maybe something that threatened your livelihood?

When you are absolutely focused on an outcome, haven't you always found a way? When you give an intense level of focus to achieve your goals, the results are inevitable. By giving focus to your goals, you are creating your future. When you focus on something intensely enough, your attention transmits energy. As an ultrarunner, moving creates energy, and in that sense, your movement is near infinite.

'Focus' is the first ingredient to any dream, while doubt can be the death of it. Doubt kills dreams because the fear of failure triggers self-doubt. Examples are thoughts of not training enough, not finishing a race, or facing danger. But what is 'failure,' exactly? In my opinion, it's whatever definition you give it. The official definition of failure is a 'lack of success' and to be a success is 'to achieve a desired aim.' Well, if you are the one aiming, then you are the one who determines if you lack success from your actions. But what if you gave failure a new association? What if you looked at a potential 'failure' as a learning opportunity? This way, if you do not reach a desired outcome, but you learn from the experience, then it's far from a failure. Also, remember this: excuses are the kryptonite to your dreams.

As I mentioned, a few years ago, I was traveling towards the beach for a summer vacation on the east coast of the United States. On the way, I was dropped off 37 miles from my destination and walked from mile 28.

But since I stopped running, was this a failure? Far from it, because at that moment, I did something that changed my running career forever. Enough was enough. Like I said, I took off the GPS watch attached to my wrist and launched it as far as my arm could throw it. You see, I learned something about myself that day. That day, I learned that monitoring my time, splits, and pace while running did not motivate me – actually, they did the exact opposite. For me, checking my pace over and over again added an extra weight on my shoulders. My thought process was this: all week I work on a clock, go to appointments at set times, and go to engagements, in addition to all the many other time-set activities. With this in mind, why would I choose to be on a clock when I'm running? That is, why put a time on something I love? Running was my escape, but the watch tamed my ambitions. Running on a clock was the exact opposite of the reason I was running in the first place. When running, I enjoy the freedom, the independence, and the solitude. Not the splits, the pace, and the time. Don't get me wrong; this same demotivation might well motivate other runners. We all have our own associations and motivations. The key is to learn what your motivations are and use them to your advantage to progress as athletes in your chosen sport.

Secret Ingredient #2: Passion

Be obsessed with running, fall in love with running, do not shy away from running. Be PASSIONATE about running. When you do something that you love, have you ever noticed how fast time passes? When we take on a task with passion, time becomes a relevance lost in space while the drive to move becomes natural. When we move with drive, we feel alive. When I write and run, I lose myself in the moment, and time becomes infinite. I love running, I love writing, and I love to inspire. When I publish something and see such an incredible response, I'm instantly motivated. What motivates me most is the possibility that someone could be one step closer to achieving a personal goal very close to their hearts. If you can be passionate about running, you can give it the care and the level of energy it needs. Passion is an unbelievable force that can awaken you from even the greatest depths of your daily routine. By snapping you out of your state of lethargy, it gives you the boost that you need to move through a training program towards your next finish line. Stuck in a slump? Get passionate. Blocked by limiting beliefs? Get passionate. Questioning your abilities? Get passionate. If you run and are reading this, chances are you are passionate about running, whether you realize it or not. Passion gives you certainty in your capabilities and an immeasurable amount of drive. The results can become effortless, in a way. Think about the motivation you get when you *want* to do something, versus when you *have* to do something. If YOU want to run those miles, then YOU will run those miles.

Secret Ingredient #3: Faith

Uncertain if the distance is possible? We will all experience some level of uncertainty in running, no matter how focused we are. But understand this: understand that it is absolutely possible. As runners, we will all feel uncertain at times and be forced to take risks. The level of risk is up to us. So if risk is bound to happen, if risk is unavoidable, if risk is inevitable, then shouldn't we risk believing in ourselves? When we contemplate taking a chance on ourselves, faith will help us move forward. Faith gives us that level of certainty to combat hesitation. Sure, we do not know where it comes from; this is a given. But just like all of the most significant figures throughout time, you must decide to have it anyway. Have faith in your abilities, in your strength, and in your courage.

Standing at the starting line of my first 100-mile ultramarathon, I was completely uncertain if I could cover a distance of such magnitude. But this was true before every new distance. I had some level of uncertainty before my first 50k, 50 miles, 100K, my first 100 miles, and the first time I broke 100 miles. Sure, there was a level of uncertainty, but I had faith in myself. With faith, I was able to stand at the starting line with my chin up on every race day morning, ready to tackle what I considered impossible at the time. These were all risks I decided to take with faith in my abilities to finish. You need faith, in the ultra world, and that's why faith is the final ingredient.

When running ultramarathons, we learn a lot about running and at the same time, we learn a lot about ourselves. We run many different ultramarathons in our lives, both literally and metaphorically. I've run diligently and methodically at some times, and at other times, I've run spontaneously and unprepared. Either way, you can always focus on goals, drive with passion, and put faith in the outcomes.

It's most important that you run the way you love to run, whichever way you feel pulled towards. If beating a PR provides you with significance, then go for a new time. If the distance motivates you, then go after those long miles. If it's a sense of community that sparks your interests, then join a running club. We get so caught up in what we think we should do, but we must listen to our own bodies and think for ourselves. When running and living as who you truly are, focus, passion, and faith will come naturally. It moves you to your next finish line, and it will drive you to something more, more of who you really are: a RUNNER!

CHAPTER 17

Thank You Ultrarunning

Before leaving you off on the road to ultramarathon success, let's touch on an important subject. The subject I'm talking about is by far one of the most powerful tools when we run, and in life in general. The tool I'm referring to is 'gratification.'

Chasing a time, a particular qualifying event, or placement, are typical running practices. But, for some, what motivates us at the starting line can be the death of us before ever reaching the finish. For some, it leaves us chasing an external outcome with our mind focused on the finish line. I've run fixated on the finish line, chasing a time I was expected to run or a place I was supposed to be in. But I've also run with gratitude for the now, for the moment, and for myself. And you know what? Gratification trumps expectation tenfold. What can you be grateful for when running? Be grateful for your health, your bones, and your muscles. Be grateful for the trails, the earth, and the weather. Be grateful for your fellow runners, the volunteers, and the support of your family and friends. Be grateful for the time, your love for running, and the shoes on your feet. Be grateful for anything and everything. When you are feeling grateful, it's almost impossible to feel bad! So when you add it to a sport where intense physical and mental pain is a guarantee, gratification will help you along the way.

So be grateful for the freedom that you can walk out of your door and be and do anything you want. Be grateful that since you have created your limiting beliefs, you can also destroy them! Only then can you achieve even your most significant goals. Perhaps you could even run an ultramarathon!

So before we conclude this book, I would like to say thank you to ultramarathon running. A sport that not only has changed my life but quite possibly saved it as well.

It's sure been one enduring and adventurous ride. Although it's been a relatively short time thus far, my gratitude is abundant. I give thanks through those leg-pounding, quad-crushing, mind-bending, never-ending miles. Ultrarunning teaches us many lessons about ourselves. The type of lessons that only surface from the struggle we face when running ultra-distances. My appreciation goes beyond belief as I tie up my running shoes before each new race. When I look back on my journey, standing at each new starting line, I say thanks. I give thanks for the health in my body, the determination in my mind, and the faith in my soul. Gratitude opens the door to a much higher quality of running and a much higher quality of life. In a world where tomorrow is never promised, I thank ultrarunning for teaching me to run in the now. Living in the now is life because life is only available at the present moment.

Thank you for the certainty you provide with every new run. When the day goes haywire and the nights become hectic, I can always count on a long run to clear my mind. When you allow significant time for yourself, you can then give much more to others. In turn, I've become a better dad, husband, writer, and a better individual.

We are all creatures of habit and ultrarunning has brought a daily fix of accomplishment into my life. It's ironic how an extremely discomforting sport can provide so much comfort. I always know where my running shoes are, my many, many running shoes and the trails are always just around the corner. Deep down inside, I know as I approach the starting line, one way or another, I will move my feet forward to that finish. I thank you for that.

Thank you for the adventure and the surprise you bring into my life. Variety makes us feel alive. The unique experiences during these exceptionally long runs have been interesting, to say the least. For the people I've run into, and I mean literally run into, and the wild animals I've run from. To the mouthfuls of mud and the toenails I've lost. For the wrong trails I've taken and the new trails to come, I thank you for the challenges I face. These challenges have provided me with the opportunity to strengthen my abilities. In ultramarathons, you can expect the unexpected. Can you feel the adventure? I thank you for that.

Most of my life has been on the move, always on my feet. I've always been attracted to enduring and action-oriented tasks while achieving growth. I never knew why this was. I still don't. But I'm thankful for discovering a platform where my strengths can be brought to light, a place they can be shared, a place I can call home. I thank you for that.

Growth is the way of life. Everything around you is growing, from the trees in the forest to the bacteria in your body. If you are not moving forward, then you are moving backward. Ultrarunners of all shapes and sizes are pushing past their limits all the time. This encourages others to challenge the impossible. We all inspire each other to go harder and to move farther than ever before. In ultrarunning, our growth will provide us with a sense of fulfillment as human beings. I thank you for that.

Although we live and take care of ourselves, life is ultimately about each other. Ultrarunning allows us to share our unique experiences and to learn from one another. We learn what works well for ourselves and what does not. It places you in one amazingly unique community. A community where anyone is welcome if they are up for the challenge. I thank you for all the great athletes I've learned from along the way and for all the knowledge I've been able to pass on to others. Although I'm nowhere close to my final running destination, I'm thankful for the journey I'm on. We can see adversity as stressful, or we can see it as a chance to improve. I thank you for that.

From the extended periods upon our feet, our bodies become stronger as we expand by demand. I thank you for the health and vitality I've achieved, both directly and indirectly, from ultrarunning. The amount of energy gained for the day from constantly running has become abundant. Although this amount of stress on the body is not always healthy, the dietary and lifestyle changes I've made have been amazing. I thank you for that.

Deep down beyond the pain in my legs, I focus on what I'm grateful for. Like I mentioned before, when we are feeling grateful, it's almost impossible to feel bad. So in a sport where intense physical and mental pain is guaranteed, gratitude can help you along the way.

CONCLUSION

I remember the first step I took as a new runner and the last step before finishing my first ultramarathon. At the time, it sure seemed like a whole lot of ground to cover. But in ultrarunning, you come to realize that it's never been about the race to finish. It's always been about the journey to travel. You will have bad days and good days, slow runs and fast runs, tough races and easy races. But you will only have one journey. Sure, the path may get challenging, but isn't that true for all roads less traveled? Remember, when you finish an ultramarathon, you enter the 0.1% club. Only 0.1%, or one-tenth of one percent, of the US population, has completed an ultramarathon. If it were easy, everyone would do it.

When we are new to ultrarunning, somewhere past the marathon is where the real challenge begins. Here is where the real pain sets in, both physically and mentally. Here is when your mind tells you to STOP! "Come on, what's the point?" "Why are you running this thing anyway?" "Who cares if you quit?" "You gave a good effort, let's call it a day!" But know this: the same wall that blocks disappointment is the same wall that blocks triumph. The same wall that blocks failure is the same wall that blocks success. And the same wall that blocks our regret is the same wall that blocks our dreams. Luckily, the moment your body gives up is the exact moment when your heart gives more. It tells you to run for something greater, something worth the pain and worth the struggle. It reminds you of those long months, those tiring days, and those weekend sacrifices. It reminds you how bad you want it and how bad you DESERVE it. Yes, running an ultramarathon for the first time is challenging, but yes, it's possible. If you keep pushing yourself and you break past the fear and self-doubt, guess what? The dynamics change completely! All of a sudden, as you move forward, you don't just run to the finish line, you gravitate towards it! Then you reach the end where those last few miles feel like you're flying as the finish line comes into vision – and suddenly, all of those questions of "is it worth it?" and "what's the point?" instantly disintegrate. They disappear along with all the other excuses that tried stopping you from reaching this victorious moment. And then it happens, you cross the finish line, and suddenly, it all makes sense. Suddenly you come to realize that you didn't just run an ultramarathon to better your running, you ran it to better your life!

So let me be the first to congratulate you. You have just taken the hardest step towards achieving any goal. You have taken the FIRST step. Deciding and getting started with running an ultramarathon is the hardest step of all. Now it's time to apply this new-found knowledge. Remember, knowledge isn't power, knowledge with ACTION is power. When you learn something and then apply it to your life, that's when you change your circumstances, that's when you change your life.

I am super-excited you've taken the first steps towards your new running goals with The Ultramarathon Guide as your roadmap. I sincerely hope that I was able to help you understand the best ways to become an ultramarathon runner.

Yes, The Ultramarathon Guide is your road map to finishing the ultramarathon of your dreams. So train hard, train smart, and most importantly of all, never EVER give up.

Thank you, and enjoy every minute of your new life as an ultramarathon runner!

Printed in Great Britain
by Amazon